THE 10 COMMANDMENTS OF ENERGY MASTERY

The 10 Commandments of Energy Mastery

Creating Personal Power & Freedom

VICKI ADRIANNE

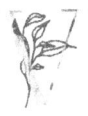

Given the bold title of this book and the incredible contents you are about to read and integrate into your life, remember this:

> *Love the Lord your God with all your heart and with all your soul and with all your mind.*
> *This is the first and greatest commandment.*
> *And the second is like it: Love your neighbor as yourself.'*
> Matthew 22: 37-39

Copyright

Rise in Power; The Ten Commandments of Energy Mastery. Creating Personal Power and Freedom

Copyright © 2021 by Vicki Adrianne. All rights reserved. No part of this publication may be reproduced, distributed, or transmitted in any form or by any means-electronic, mechanical, photocopy, recording or any other- except for brief quotations in printed reviews, without prior written permission of the author.

Vickiadrianne.com
Paperback ISBN: 978-1-7777472-1-3
Digital ISBN: 978-1-7777472-0-6
First Edition
Canada

Disclaimer

The ideas and concepts in this book are based on my experience and what has and has not worked for me. While I hope this book provides valuable guidance, I cannot know the full details of any reader's personal situation.

This book is designed to provide information that the author believes to be accurate, but it is sold with the understanding that the author is not offering individualized advice tailored to any individual's particular needs. The author disclaims any responsibility for any liability, loss or risk, personal or otherwise which is incurred as a direct or indirect consequence of the use and application of any of the contents of this book.

The information in this book is not intended or implied to be a substitute for professional medical advice, diagnosis, or treatment. All content in this book is for general information purposes only and not offered as medical or psychological advice, guidance, or treatment. Please see a medical professional if you need help with depression, illness, or have any concerns whatsoever. All information is provided on an as-is basis. You are solely responsible for your own choices and actions.

What people say about working with Vicki

"I had the most amazing experience with Vicki! She uncovered for me, in one hour, what many other coaches, holistic therapists, and medical experts were unable to. It was the most eye-opening experience; one that has put me on a path to healing, self-awareness, and self-love. I am eternally grateful, will return for additional sessions and highly recommend her services. She has a gift that goes beyond anything words could begin to describe." -Melanie M., St. John's NFLD

"You have helped me let go of past memories that kept me bound; and I am now able to live in the present." -Melanae

"Vicki is the lighthouse guiding us through our fears and anxieties; through treacherous waters of trauma, shedding her light and love on the darkest of nights so we can sail safely to the shore." -Amanda Muis

"I will look back on our valuable work together and know that you had a massive impact on my life. The changes I see in myself are wonderful." -Rob

Vicki Holleman is truly tuned into the higher realms and able to help you see how to embody the energies you need at this time. She is a great seer and knower of the deeper truth of what is wanting to happen through you. -Daniel John Hanneman, Founder, Academy for Invincible Healers.

Vicki, Please continue to share your gift as the world will be altered by it. -Jill Prescott, Spiritual Badass

I had a healing session with Vicki Holleman and am grateful for her skill as a healer. I feel so much lighter after having been expertly guided by Vicki to let go of and clear some areas of my life that previously felt overly thick and heavy. It's a week later now and my world continues to open up in ways that are new and very much in line with my goals. Thanks Vicki. -Norman Mann, Certified Hypnotherapist

"My connection to God has strengthened and the dark cloud has gone away. Thanks Vicki! You are the real deal and you are a blessing to all those that come your way. -Tarek Bibi, Founder of Infinity Healing

Vicki's warm, open energy allowed me to feel safe to express myself during our session, which enable truth to come through in ways that surprised me. I felt completely comfortable speaking with her as she held space for the energy within to be seen and unravel. I would highly recommend Vicki to anyone in search of unbiased insight, and loving support. Whether one is going through major life changes or just seeking gently guidance around an emotional issue. I felt truly seen and met..it was a wonderful experience! -J. McGregor

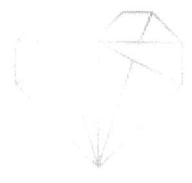

Acknowledgements

This book was in the making for a few years and I am forever grateful to those who have helped shape and form this publication.

First, to my teachers, coaches, mentors and guides for helping me find the light in myself and encouraging me to shine it. Thank you from the core of my heart.

Thank you to my editors, Lynn, Syl, and Donna. This book would have been a mess without your insight, keen eyes, and willingness to help.

Thank you to my clients for trusting me as your guide. You inspire me with your courage every day.

Contents

Introduction   1

Part One: Your Foundation   9

1	Cultivate Gentle Awareness	10
2	Nourish Thyself	31
3	Love Thyself	66
4	Follow Thy Heart	86

Part Two: Embody All You Are Made To Be   113

5	Own Your Boundaries	114
6	Love Your Body	145
7	Breathe and Meditate	155

Part Three: Ongoing Maintenance 171

8 Forgive and Let Go 172

9 Take Action 195

10 Never Give Up 223

Conclusion 243

Introduction

After choosing faith and trust amidst my darkest moment, I pulled myself out of victimhood by deciding not to be a victim and dedicated my life to Truth (with a capital T). Over eight years I went from a place of rock bottom; homeless, bankrupt, and afraid of the dark, to thriving in a way I never imagined possible. Along the way, on my journey back to my true self, I learned so much that I began sharing with others in my one-on-one practice and group workshops.

Teaching energy mastery is my passion. I won't be here forever and I want to leave a legacy of empowerment, and I feel it is needed in a world of constant change. I want to teach what I have learned about being deeply connected to your true self so it can guide you forward, and give you impactful tools to clear whatever is in the way of your clarity and confidence.

What I share in this book are the essential keys to energy mastery. Having shared them with hundreds of people I have witnessed the magnificent shifts these tools and practices can create in one's life. From overcoming lifelong labels, to manifesting loving committed relationships, to increasing health and energy so you can get done what you have always wanted to do.

I never thought I had it in me to write a book like this, but with the right knowledge and truly listening to my heart for guidance, here it is, in your hands. I know as you read it you will have many Eureka! moments. You may feel triggered at times, but don't fret, there are tools on how to deal with being triggered. Don't shy away from the triggers, they can be catalysts for awareness, healing, and mastery.

When your heart is engaged as much as your mind you integrate lessons faster and deeper so you truly reap the rewards of your life experience. Allowing your heart to be fully open in your life, you can no longer hide from what is being called out in you, your truth, beauty, and greatness. As you surrender again and again to the path of your heart, you illuminate your whole self, becoming stronger, a brighter light as all that blocks the light fades away.

I believe in the healing force of love. Even in the midst of death and decay, which is a natural part of life, as is the grief and sorrow that comes with it, love is present as a healing force. No matter what you have been through, you can learn the lessons and heal to wholeness. I believe in the power of the breath and the truth of the heart.

Through each of the chapters that follow you will be gaining more and more awareness about who you are, and how to become all you can be. This stems from an open heart and clarity of body, mind, and spirit which you will gain as you read and practice the tools and exercises in this book.

Please get yourself a journal to write your aha's and insights. There will be some journal prompts throughout the book to help you integrate all you are learning. This book isn't only a quick and easy read. It is meant to impact you profoundly if you open your heart and mind as you take it in.

My intention in writing this book is to help you build a foundation for truly stepping into and owning your power from the moment you open it until the day you leave the planet. As you read I invite you to consider that personal power and energy mastery are less about control and more about surrender. Surrender to the divine presence that is you at your core, resting deep within your heart.

The book starts with physical practices of energy mastery and then goes deeper into the mind, heart, soul, and spirit.

In Part One you will learn the foundational principles and practices of energy mastery.

In chapter one, you will learn the scientific and spiritual truth that energy is everything and gain insight and tools to cultivate awareness that will amplify your mastery skills. With this awareness, you can use your energy for all the good you desire to experience in life, even when surrounded by present-day challenges.

Chapter two covers the fundamentals of how to use food as fuel for energy and see where you've been duped by big business into believing misinformation about what is healthy and why. You'll learn to see your body as the temple it is and to feed yourself from love instead of self-hate or bodily control. You'll learn the basics of your body's different systems and how to support your optimal health for natural, vibrant energy.

Chapter three will teach you how loving yourself will help you love others more. You'll become aware of your self-talk and learn new effective ways to create supportive thought patterns that lift you up instead of tear you down. You'll learn the dirty secret behind the Secret and how to turn your heart's desires into real-world expressions and experiences for personal growth.

In the final chapter of this section, you will learn tools to truly listen to your heart and take action on where it is calling you. You'll see how following your heart leads to fulfillment and graceful living. After reading this chapter you will be able to trust your intuition and act on it, and make peace between your head and your heart.

Part two will help you embody the foundation to become grounded and present in your life right now.

In chapter five you will claim your energetic authority through boundaries. You will see how boundaries are critical to energy mastery and how to enforce them gracefully and in a way that feels natural. Boundaries help you stay connected to your truth and after reading this chapter you will have a new understanding of how this works in your body and how to communicate and maintain boundaries in your life and relationships.

Chapter six will show you exactly how looking radiant and feeling good go together. Exercise isn't just for the body, it's for all of you. You will integrate your mind and spirit with physical exercise and learn to use your ego to enhance your health.

Chapter seven will help you raise your clarity and confidence through breath and meditation. It will help you increase your focus so you can achieve your goals. You will also learn the art of using the breath to open your heart so you can be powerful, present, and continually aligning yourself from the inside out.

Part three will help you with ongoing maintenance and integration so you can live authentically in your life after you finish this book.

Chapter eight will show how letting go of the past raises your energy, impacting your life and your relationships. You will learn how to express yourself fully even if you've held yourself back for years or even decades. You'll discover how all emotions, regardless of if you've previously labeled them as good or bad are a part of your wholeness. You will receive tools to nurture and protect your energy as you grow in your authentic self.

Overcoming obstacles is an ongoing part of life and in chapter nine you'll learn how to work with your primal fears to move forward when you feel stuck. You'll learn the energetic truth behind vision boards, see the significance of a positive attitude and how to have true goals, and build habits that lead to achievement.

And finally, in chapter ten, you will integrate how to have the kind of faith and trust that moves you forward. You will discover how to set up your environment for success. You will see how often you might get in your own way and how to stop holding yourself back.

You will finish with a cementing reminder and life lesson on how to use gratitude, enthusiasm, laughter, and celebration to enjoy life more.

The illustrations in this book are pictures taken directly out of my journal. I am no artist but I think they are good visuals to help you fully understand the concepts. I hope they help you integrate what you are learning.

Happy reading!

Part One: Your Foundation

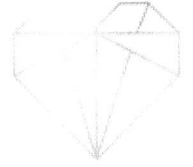

Chapter 1

Cultivate Gentle Awareness

*Energy is Everything
and
Everything is Energy*

The statement "energy is everything" is true, however, it doesn't mean much if you don't have awareness. Awareness is the first step to energy mastery and any kind of healing that will take place in your life.

When you become aware of your energy, and how it reflects into the world, you can make small or big changes that will lead to greater prosperity, reduced stress, improved health, and better relationships with others and yourself. I will share many tools in this book to gain insight into yourself and how to roll with the ups and downs of life with ease and lasting inner peace.

The first question I often hear is, "How do I gain awareness?"

To begin, simply ask for awareness. Ask yourself or your intuition, ask a higher power of your belief (whether that's God, Universe, Your highest self), ask to be given the gift of awareness of your energy and how it is impacting your life. Your energy is always flowing, it is the life force animating your body. As we move through life we experience times of fear which create contraction or barriers which limit our natural energy flow. When not addressed these contractions can stay in the body and nervous system creating blocks that prevent us from fully expressing ourselves, feeling fully confident, or re-arranging our behaviors to avoid triggering the past fear the block is rooted in. As you continue reading this book you will dive deeper into this and gain even more awareness and tools to help you master your energy and live your best life regardless of seeming "outer" circumstances or past experiences.

"Awareness is separate from thinking."

Bill Clum

Cultivating awareness helped me go from literally being afraid of the dark, to unearthing and releasing my true self who was hidden in darkness. I am no longer afraid to shine my light! Now I help others move trapped emotions and release themselves from fear and pain. Do yourself a favor and read this book to the end. I promise to give you tons of information and help, then if you want more after there are plenty of ways to continue. You are not alone! ***Energy mastery is a skillset and a lifestyle that has a profound impact not only in your life but in the lives of all those you encounter.*** You will see how as you read on.

Begin right now. Ask for awareness every day for the next week. Asking for awareness is a great tool if you ever feel stuck or want more awareness about what is happening in your life.

> Ask, and it shall be given you; seek, and ye shall find; knock, and it shall be opened unto you:
> For every one that asketh receiveth; and he that seeketh findeth; and to him that knocketh it shall be opened.
> Matthew 7:7-8

When you ask for awareness you will begin to see where your energy is entangled in your mind and energy body, as well as the entanglements you have with other people, old stories, and ideas. With this awareness, you can begin to gain the ultimate life-directing clarity and confidence as you live your life from your authentic self.

Beginning with asking yourself and the Divine for awareness leads to this path that you will never want to leave. The path of your true heart, your true power, your true love. This path will take you far beyond what you could have imagined is possible for you. Take a moment to reflect now on what might be possible for you if you had access to your inner power and went through your day with clarity, inner wisdom, and confidence. You can write this in your journal or simply close your eyes and take a few deep breaths and imagine the possibilities...

Now that you have some insight into what is possible, let's touch base on why you may not already be there. What is it that prevents you from shining your light fully, being free and expressive of your true heart's desires? What prevents you from mastering yourself so you maintain your energy, clarity, and confidence every day?

There are many reasons, and each of them can be worked through to get to where you want to be. While you will be focusing on the positive and how to be more positive in every moment, we need to acknowledge the so-called "negative"; the shadow aspect that everyone has. These shadows or hidden aspects of yourself can be due to your past experiences that have colored your perceptions, ways of being, and current ability to step beyond your comfort zone. They may come from traumatic experiences locked into your body and mind which can wreak havoc on your ultimate happiness and expressive freedom.

You cannot deny your shadow. We all have one. Awareness is what allows you to not let the shadow-self take over and ruin what you are living for. Awareness is key as shadows can show up when you least expect or want them to, often causing rifts in relationships and sabotaging the results you are hoping for.

The shadow is the hidden part of yourself you like to pretend doesn't exist and when it shows up you can feel confused about the way a specific situation unfolded, or like you've lost control. As human beings, we all have shadow aspects to ourselves we can heal and integrate when we begin with gentle awareness. My shadow shows up like a whiny baby or an angry teenager. If I'm getting frustrated but pretend everything is ok I get even more frustrated. Yet, if I honor the shadow part of me that needs to vent or release the valve of pent-up energy I can set a timer for five to ten minutes, get the energy of frustration out through healthy emotional expression, and then am back to normal.

Growing up I thought "if I am a good girl in the eyes of others and get good grades my life will be easy as an adult." Ha! It turned out being a good girl with good grades wasn't enough for the totality of me. Me, including my shadow, had an entire range of ways of being that wanted to come out and play- the rebel in particular.

Rebels aren't bad when directed properly, they can break the norms and create breakthroughs in all areas of life. Jesus was a rebel, going against the strict traditions of the day to offer greater love and forgiveness in life. But without direction, rebels can become destructive. My inner rebel moved to far eastern Russia on a youth exchange program at the young age of eighteen. Then, after university, moved across Canada. She was hungry for big experiences and went out and got them. When things became too still during my rebellious phases and I didn't know about energy management, let alone mastery, my shadow took over. All the emotions under the surface would come up and out like a burst of anger at a boyfriend or having a "poor me" victim mentality with myself and others. I did not know inner wisdom or how to flow with and release the buried emotion, and how to center and ground myself in my heart to begin again from within.

Becoming aware of my shadow, the parts of my subconscious that my ego-mind doesn't want to acknowledge, fully accepting and expressing all of me, including my shadow aspects, has led to being able to be with all of myself with compassion, and continue to grow without the burden of making myself wrong for not being "the good girl", "successful according to society", or anything else other than all of what and who I am.

Casting light on shadows through gentle awareness helps you recognize that they served a purpose for you. The purpose of a shadow may be to protect you, help you learn from past mis-takes (mistakes are just mis-takes), and experience gratitude for how unique your life is. You can then gratefully integrate and learn the message your shadow has and lovingly call more of your divine light into your life as you learn new ways of being that feel good and put you on track to fulfill your desires. You can learn more about shadows by checking out any of Debbie Ford's work or anyone else you resonate with.

Remember, you are whole. Inherent wholeness fulfills desires, naturally. Wholeness is accepting every part of you unconditionally. What is it that prevents you from experiencing wholeness? During the first part of your life, you are learning so much about the outer physical world and its workings you often forget the inner world. Other's voices become dominant in your psyche and you may have developed a loud inner critic. The inner critic is a voice that tries to keep you in check (ie. locked in a box marked "appropriate according to society"). "Make sure you are doing everything perfectly," it says, or it tells you you are not good enough, perhaps even that you are a terrible person. The inner critic wracks you with unnecessary guilt about all sorts of topics from grades or income, to your body, to how clean your house is. The inner critic ALWAYS takes you out of the present moment and into your head.

Take a few deep breaths right now and remember your heart.
Stop. Breathe.
Count backward from ten and drop into your heart, breathing deeply.
   10
   9
   8
   7
   6
   5
   4
   3
   2
   1

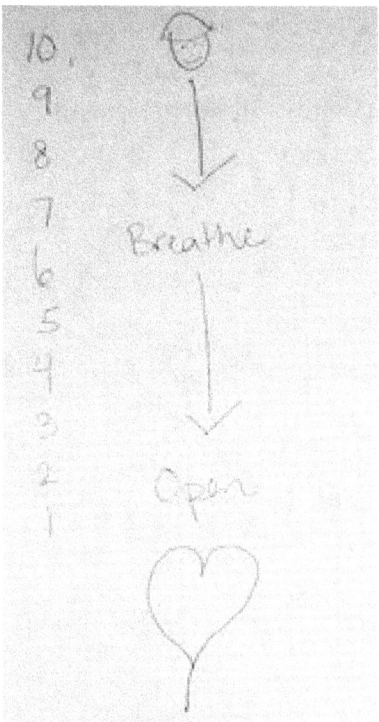

Notice a difference? You will be coming back to your heart often in this book.

Your shadows and inner critic may have been getting stirred up as you read about them. Always come back to your heart. The more light of awareness is shone on the inner critic and other aspects of the psyche including shadows, behaviors, beliefs, thoughts, or actions you want to shift, the more you become aware of how they impact you. Awareness breeds more awareness and when you lovingly inquire what is there for you from the heart space, through this "dropping into your heart" countdown, the faster you integrate or release what has been holding you back.

The skill of self-awareness has me recognize different aspects of myself, including my shadows, as they come up to be integrated with my whole Self. From my inner child to my rebellious teenager, to my higher/wiser self, I can witness their wisdom and listen to what they need or have to offer at the moment. Sometimes they are quiet and I don't notice them for days if I don't take time to meditate and breathe. If I don't notice them right away I usually get a physical symptom like bloating, a sore neck, or foot cramp for example. I find when I take time to breathe into the area with the symptom there is a message that comes through the unfolding of pent-up energy that manifested as the symptom in the first place. The symptom is a message from the body to go within. Symptoms are often a reflection of unmet needs.

The next time you feel tense, first take notice that you are tense. Begin to breathe deeply, connecting with your lungs and the oxygen flowing through your blood and bring your attention to the tension and invite it to release. Once the initial tension is gone ask specific areas of tension if there is a message for you.

Take the time to deeply listen.

You may feel an emotion surface such as sadness. Allow it to come up and be felt. Breathe deeply, having a compassionate inner dialogue as you set the emotion free and integrate any message it had for you. Be grateful you now know the message. Journaling can help you integrate the lesson.

This process, used as a tool in your energy mastery toolbox, can lift a weight off your shoulders. Please take note of it and perhaps do a practice around now and I'll introduce you to several other techniques and practices to empower you throughout the book.

*

A note on trauma and post-traumatic stress disorder:

When you experience trauma and suffer from PTSD it can throw you off balance for days, weeks, months, and even years if not addressed properly. Trauma is common and it's important to be open about it without shaming it or blaming the circumstance that caused it, or blaming yourself. Instead, you can see it as something that happened that you can effectively address through proper care.

When left unexamined and untreated trauma and PTSD can lock into the nervous system, brain, and psyche and affect your whole life from how you feel in every moment, and that impacts the long-term outcomes of your life. This book does not claim to heal trauma and PTSD although having been through it myself I know the tools in this book have helped me and I will offer some insight. If you are suffering please get qualified medical, psychological, and alternative help that resonates with you and do everything you can to find your balance and peace again.

*

Your past experiences have impacted you. From being a baby until today, right now where you sit with this book in your hands. Your past experiences shape how you see the world, how safe you feel, what you are willing to do and not do, how you enter into relationships of all sorts, how you handle your money, and how you take care of your health.

Everyone is unique and two people could have the same experience yet perceive it completely differently, therefore, creating a different effect in their lives. I will cover lots of examples throughout this book to show you how sneaky some of these ways of being can be and how to overcome them so you keep reaching for your goals and evolving into the expression of the magnificence you are created to be.

I will share some processes in this book about how you can take a disempowering experience and turn it into fuel for your empowered life. First, it's important to acknowledge sometimes you may not even be aware of how your past is affecting you. As you continue reading, open your mind and heart and be willing to look, do the self-inquiry, and do the work to uncover areas of your life that no longer serve you. Each behavior and experience you have been living has served you in some way but if that is no longer true there are ways to let them go, re-frame them, and integrate them into your wholeness. When you do this, you create space for more good energy, awareness, and mastery to become the foundation of your everyday life. This creates the epic long-term results you desire, whether it is a simple life or an extravagant one.

What you desire is already a part of you, but you need to clear what's holding you back so you can get it. As you continue reading this book you will gain insights that can lead the way to your ultimate fulfillment, which by the way is already right here, right now!

Remember to Breathe!
The breath is your key to feeling free from the inside out in this moment.

When you don't learn to master your energy and heal your past, the energy you carry around and circulate every day can become stagnant. Ultimately you want to keep your energy fresh and moving but without the energy mastery principles in this book, you can become bogged down with old energy, and often the energy of others you knowingly or unknowingly carry. You share energy with those you have intimate relations with, family members, people you serve at work, people you encounter in public, and even total strangers you walk by on the street. You know this to be true and have probably noticed certain people carry "positive" or "negative" energy. You can feel lighter when in the presence of light energy people, and heavier after a time with a negative person or even an "energy vampire", someone who seems to suck the life force right out of you. At the end of this book, you will know how to be one of the lighter energy people, avoid or not get drained by vampires, and even help light others up with your presence because you have set free the light within.

As you begin to live from your heart, from the inside out, your whole world becomes illuminated.

One of the core elements in this book is the idea of self-expression. If you repress or suppress your true authentic self you become stagnant as your inner light cannot get out without being filtered. Over time this can lead to depression and other ailments. It is also what leads to the creation and perpetuation of your shadow aspects.

Repression
+
Suppression
=
Depression

As a society, we are coming to the end of an era of suppression. Perhaps you too have held back due to fear of persecution, abuse, and even simply being seen in your full light. Suppressing your expression is causing excess energy to store and stagnate in your energy body, sometimes manifesting as physical illness or disease. When you start letting these old energies out, begin verbalizing your desires, and communicating from a place of inner truth, the freedom you experience is brilliant. It's not some hype from a motivational speaker (although they can be awesome), but true inner strength and freedom which feels so good that you have no choice but to align your words and actions with it!

Seek and find sacred spaces held by those who have done the work before you and you will shed the immeasurable weight of previous suppression to find your alignment. A sacred space can be a specific place dedicated to spiritual practice such as a private nook or room with an altar full of things meaningful to you. Or it can mean the energy of a place which may be held by non-judgmental teachers or guides who help you find your truth. I have an altar space in my home with a bright window, a plant that belonged to my grandmother to keep me connected to my roots, crystals that were gifts from my mentors, and my journal to help me meaningfully process the unfolding of my life. I also seek out sacred spaces with my mentors. Having supported them in a few workshops I have witnessed them sit in a room where a meditation is to be held and ask for higher guidance, pray, and set their intentions for the meditation or workshop they are about to hold. I also do similar practices before any workshop or session I host to create the "sacred space". You being in your power now will be a practice and an unfolding. In this process, know divine love is always there, calling and guiding you forward.

Another way your light gets dulled is when you give your power and energy away. This is common with caring people who want to help others. Thank God for these amazing folks but if you are one of them, please take care of yourself. You will have more energy to truly give in a way that serves, and people will notice.

One day, as I was beginning to write this book, I had a conversation with an elderly lady in the hospital. She was awaiting a large bone graft on her right leg, unable to get out of bed. She was kind but deeply troubled because she felt she was at the end of her life with no one there for her.

She told me, "I gave and gave everything I ever had in my life. My time, my money, oh so much money, my energy, all to help others. I forgot to take care of myself first."

I did my best to listen with compassion and offer some love by keeping my heart open in service.

Then she continued, "Oh how I regret that! Laying here now, like this, I can see how I can be a giver and supporter of others but how much better it could have been if I had started within and given from a full cup!"

I agreed self-care is paramount, reflecting on my own experiences in life. Mid-memory, she jumped in, her voice stronger than it had been during our conversation.

Emphatically, she said, "Promise me you will take care of yourself first! Promise me!"

I promised.

I know when I care for myself first I can serve from a full and overflowing cup of peaceful presence and love.

In my life I used to be a total people pleaser, trying to make everyone around me happy and attempting to be seen as a good girl. When this didn't work I turned my upset and anxiety about it towards myself which turned into negative self-talk, eating disorders, and I eventually became so disconnected from my voice that I gave my power away to all sorts of people and institutions which left me at rock bottom. In 2010 I found myself homeless, bankrupt, and living in fear after giving myself away to a narcissist who sucked the life force out of me. After hitting rock bottom I dedicated my life to truth and healing which has led to uncovering the wisdom in this book and the development of my work with others.

Mastering your energy requires being connected to your center at all times. And when you feel off-center, being able to quickly and easily reconnect there. You will learn in the coming pages many ways to do this and different tools to reset your energy when you are feeling down, exhausted, or off-balance. I am not suggesting you don't feel the full range of your emotions and pretend to be balanced, which is called spiritual bypassing. My goal is to offer you effective solutions that have long-lasting results in your well-being.

While you don't need to learn everything, you do need tools and you do need to get support. As a human being, you are designed to live in harmony with others, and when you are on the path to greatness the more support you have the better! Whether you join groups with people who are of similar mind and heart, on the growth path, or you hire a coach it's all going to help.

Never be afraid to ask for help from someone you trust, who has a good reputation, who can see things objectively and guide you to your center and back to your path when you've gotten temporarily "lost". (Your heart always knows the way, we'll cover self-trust in chapter six). Going to events is a great way to stay social, learn new things, expand your perspective and social circle. Don't be afraid to invest in yourself, even if it's twenty dollars to go to that networking event one day. I've invested at least $50,000 in my growth and development up to this point in my life and I don't regret a single penny. It wasn't always easy but kept me focused on my drive and vision, and since I am all-in financially and otherwise, there was no room to turn back. I am fully committed and have clarity about my intention to grow, develop and expand myself.

Clarity is defined as freedom from indistinctness or ambiguity. It is when everything about a particular situation comes into focus. This is when you can let your "Yes" be your yes and your "No" be your no.

CLARITY = POWER

When you have clarity, you can access your true vision with ease and when you have that, every one of your steps forward is guided. When you have clarity, nothing and no one can hold you down from rising to your full potential. When you have clarity, your heart and mind are synchronized which reflects into your outer life as the soul force that drives your daily life. When you have clarity, you become acutely aware of when you are off balance and quickly take actions to get back to your center where your true power lies. This is the core of energy mastery. Knowing your center as who you truly are, staying in alignment, and sharing it with the world!

Energy mastery and inner peace are deeply intertwined. When you are rooted in inner peace it is near impossible to truly throw us off balance for long. Your inner peace is between you and your True Self, between you and the divine. (I am going to use the word God in this book. You may replace it with a word of your choosing. If the word God triggers you, I understand. The word God has been used to instill fear for centuries but in truth, God is good and loving and nothing to feel negativity about. You can take your power back around this word if you choose. I will share more about my own experience with this word in future chapters and I shared my full story of religious and spiritual abuse in my book Woman Rise).

You can begin to cultivate inner peace through all of the steps in this book and it begins with letting go of what others think of you and their opinions in general. Others can have their opinions but you don't need to get attached to them or involved in them. While the critical factor in developing inner peace is surrender to what is from a state of reverence and wonder, it is also important to take total responsibility for yourself. When you do this you let go of old ideas that don't work for you and open up to what is possible and own your ability to take action. This is power.

Energy is everything and everything is energy. Remember this as you continue to read. Take this book and the work here seriously, but not too seriously. Enjoy the ride as you get into the physical aspects of energy mastery and beyond, beginning with nutrition in chapter two. You've already gained awareness, now it's time for more. Keep reading...

Chapter 2

Nourish Thyself

Nutrition is a gateway drug to higher consciousness.

Your body is your temple. It houses your life force, moves your emotions, and is the vehicle through which you take actions to reach your dreams. Think about the vitality flowing through your body when it is at its best. When you are eating healthy, exercising regularly, and hydrated with clean water, you know you are doing good things for your body, mind, heart, and spirit. You also realize when you don't take care of yourself you feel it, and it is the opposite of the vibrancy you desire to feel. As you begin to own your body as your temple, you can start to make better choices. You are no longer tempted by old habits because you know what feeling good feels like, and you don't want anything less.

I used to hate my body, with such fierceness. I felt like a victim of my shape and size.

In the name of "health", I read all the tips and tricks on how to lose weight. I never considered the intricacies of the alchemical and chemical makeup of the body. It was strictly about weight and size. This led to an incredible imbalance, not only in my body but also my mind and spirit. I struggled with bloating for most of my life, often overate, had blood sugar issues, and overall felt terrible after eating, mentally, and physically.

Growing up I had terrible digestive issues that I was told are simply genetic, and had my pain dismissed as nothing serious. Over time I became addicted to sugar, had regular energy slumps, was always bloated, and couldn't figure out why. I hated my body from a very young age and suffered from anorexia and bulimia in my university years. Eventually, I became a Certified Nutritional Practitioner, and by implementing all I learned I have managed to heal my digestive concerns and love myself deeply enough to truly care for my temple from a place of love and not hatred anymore. And what a difference!

Over the past fifteen years, from being obsessed with weight loss, to becoming a raw-foodist, to barely being able to afford to eat, to becoming a certified nutritionist

I have come to learn that health, true health, cannot be measured by a scale or a measuring tape. Being an ideal weight is of course ideal, but if the rest of your life is out of whack a number or size can't save you.

If you have struggled with a poor self-image, spend lots of time filling yourself with kindness and compassion. Re-orient yourself by **listening** to what your body wants and requires for health and nourishment from a place of self-love. The body is full of wisdom and when you take time to listen to and love it, it responds positively, sharing wisdom and guidance for you to experience even greater health.

In energy mastery, there is no room for self-hate, put-downs, negative self-talk, or non-supportive comments from others. Anything other than love is either simply ignored or has the light of consciousness shone upon it to bring more love.

"***You always deserve more love, not less.***"

Matt Kahn

Your body is your temple. You are made from both stardust and the earth. The quality of food you put into your body has a massive impact on the quality and quantity of your energy and vitality! Nutrition is a huge field of work and I want to share the basics here with you. Simply put, clean pure food leads to an abundance of energy and clarity, and junk food leads to a lack of energy.

Your digestive tract runs from your mouth to your colon and does a ton of work for you every day, from chewing and breaking down food particles, to absorbing and assimilating nutrients, to excreting waste products. Your digestive system seldom rests unless you fast (ie. don't eat for a specified time of twelve hours or more). Even aside from the rest of your body, feeding the digestive system is feeding your life. If you have ever struggled with digestion I suggest getting yourself a tub of Glutamine and taking it as described on the bottle every day until it is gone. Glutamine is an amino acid that the cells of your digestive tract love. It is great for healing the digestive tract lining and supporting overall digestive health. Try it and see how you feel.

Author Michael Pollan wrote:
"*Eat food, not too much, mostly plants.*"

There are many reasons that plants should be the basis of your diet. Plants have been a major component of humanity's diet for most of history up until recently after the industrial revolution when we started eating processed foods. This shift to processed, nutrient-poor foods has a direct correlation with the obesity epidemic as well as rising rates of type two diabetes and other lifestyle-related illnesses. It is easy to get sucked into the "fast, easy, and cheap" way of eating and it's not easy to change habits. I get it, however, it can be done and if this is you, you must change, and I know you can.

Start small by adding in more real, whole plant foods, and gradually decrease your reliance on processed foods, or even better, cut out all processed junk food (even if it's labeled as healthy) immediately and you will watch your energy and clarity skyrocket! You may have to deal with cravings, mood swings, and energy imbalances for a short time while your body shifts to its new, clean, healthy fuel source but any "pain" in this case will be mostly psychological and well worth the gain of vibrant health!

Moving forward, keep your goals of feeling vibrant and healthy front and center.

Plants are abundant in nature and thanks to modern-day transportation there are endless varieties to try.

Plants come from the earth and your body is made of the earth. Your body is not made up of processed ingredients with multiple additives and preservatives, although if you continue to eat junk food you may become like that! Processed foods often contain dangerous chemicals and carcinogens in small enough amounts they don't need to be labeled but if you eat them every day imagine how it's affecting your body! It's much better to steer clear, keep your vision of yourself as healthy and vibrant, and choose what is in alignment with your vision (whole, real, plant-based foods).

I'm not arguing for veganism or vegetarianism here although that is how I have lived most of my life. There are a lot of factors that go into what is best for you. I am simply trying to make it clear that plants must be the basis of your daily food intake. Your body has an incredibly long digestive tract that can take about twenty-four hours to digest a meal depending on how dense the foods are. This is an ideal way to digest plants so you can absorb the immense amount of plant phytonutrients. On the other hand, a tiger has a short digestive tract (about five feet long) which is highly acidic to break down and eliminate the animal it ate within a few hours.

Phyto-nutrients are micro-nutrients within plant foods that are still being researched in-depth today. You are probably aware of nutrients like the minerals calcium and phosphorous, and vitamins like D, B, and C, and these are all important but there is so much more to the science of nutrition. You don't need to study this science in-depth if you don't want to. However, know when the huge dairy industry is brainwashing you into believing "Milk does a body good" because it has calcium in it they are using a single factor of goodness and avoiding all the other reasons why milk may not be the best thing for you, or the planet. It's similar to when you see a box of cereal that says it's "heart healthy!" or "high in fiber" but is also highly processed and they had to add in man-made nutrients to make it consumable. And to keep it fresh they dust the packaging with a dose of butylated hydroxytoluene, or BHT, which may have toxic effects on the liver, kidneys, and lungs (https://www.ncbi.nlm.nih.gov/m/pubmed/12396675/)

All of this processing has a massive oxidative effect on your cells. Oxidation creates free radicals, and free radicals are what cause cellular breakdown and aging. A free radical is a molecule with an unpaired electron that goes around stealing energy from other molecules creating a chain effect of oxidative damage to your cells. In this case, plants to the rescue! Plants are full of antioxidants that quell the free radicals so they can't do any more damage. Imagine if you cut out most of the food that is causing the oxidation and fill your body with antioxidants from plants instead! How great will you feel? It's like filling your body with premium fuel and letting go of any loose baggage that is slowing you down.

I will mention a few examples of how different nutrients are important to specific areas of life you may not have known. First is your bone health. You may have it in your mind that calcium is the primary factor in skeletal health. Calcium is important to your bones but what about phosphorous, boron, magnesium, and Vitamin K?

Your bones and blood have an internal buffer system to help with homeostasis (an awesome word for balance). When you drink soda it creates an acidic environment in your body, and when this happens your bones release calcium to buffer the acidity. Plants are naturally alkaline which buffers the acidity from processed junk foods as well as natural bodily processes, such as metabolism, which produce some acid. If your bodily processes create acidity naturally, you should want to fill your body with alkaline plants to keep yourself in homeostasis, balance. If you are filling your temple with junk food it will be more acidic which can lead to a decrease in bone density, muscle soreness, loss of internal nutrients, stress on the body, and has been associated with cancer and other serious illnesses.

Another example is potassium. You probably know bananas are a source of potassium and maybe growing up if you had a sore muscle your parents advised you to eat a banana. Not such bad advice. But also contained in bananas are the nutrients magnesium, folate, vitamin C, and more.

And when you have sore muscles potassium isn't the only factor involved. Other nutrients important in muscle health are clean sources of protein which are made up of amino acids and branch chain amino acids, as well as magnesium and omega-three fatty acids.

I share these brief examples to illustrate that your body is a complex and amazing work of art that requires care and attention and the importance of truly knowing your own body and not just listening to outside marketing. Use your discernment, educate yourself, work with qualified professionals, and eat mostly plants. Your body will thank you.

But how do you eat clean when the world is full of junk food and temptation is around every corner? First, you must decide that you are healthy. You must identify with yourself as a healthy person. A person who makes healthy choices, not out of depriving yourself, but because you love yourself and want to nourish and fuel your body as it supports your journey through this life. Decide, right now. Decide to be a healthy person. Healthy people truly honor themselves and this is the path you are now on.

Next, you must train yourself to the truth. The truth of who you are as a healthy person, and the truth about what healthy food is and does, and what unhealthy food is and does. Begin to see plants, fruits, and vegetables, and all unadulterated whole foods as things to keep you feeling healthy. Start to enjoy the smells and tastes of new foods if you haven't enjoyed healthy food in the past. Notice new flavors, distinguish between salty, sweet, umami, pungent, and sour flavors. Start to catch yourself when you are headed for the junk food aisle or fast food lane. Even if you notice after it's already in your belly, vow to make a better choice next time, and then next time you may notice sooner so you can stop it before it happens. Eventually, it will become second nature to make healthy choices, avoid unhealthy ones, and self-correct when you've gotten out of alignment with your core identity as healthy.

Some people think junk food is cheap and they are saving money when they buy it, but what they are doing is paying money to slowly poison themselves. See junk and highly processed foods as things difficult to digest, therefore weighing your energy down. Familiarize yourself with some food additives and what they can do to you.

Here are a couple of examples:
Tartrazine: Primarily used as Yellow Food coloring, neurotoxin linked to behavioral problems in children. Possible carcinogen (linked to cancer).
High Fructose Corn Syrup: Used as a sweetener in many processed foods, linked to weight gain and diabetes.

Speaking of high fructose corn syrup, avoid added sugars like your life depends on it- it does!

Now I'm not perfect and sometimes indulge but when I do I truly allow myself to enjoy the full experience and then when I'm fully satisfied I am right back to my healthy, plant-based, antioxidant-rich lifestyle diet. I know this can be difficult especially when your friends and family members aren't on board but stay true to you, eventually, you will have more of an influence on them than they have on you, stick to it, and remind yourself who you are, healthy, vibrant, and free. As you choose a healthier lifestyle you will also resonate at this level and attract new people into your life who share this core identity and want to support you with your healthy choices. You might find local plant-based groups, new healthy restaurants, delicious recipes, and learn all sorts of new things related to a healthy vibrant lifestyle.

Now let's talk about macronutrients. Macronutrients are fat, carbohydrates, and protein. Many people know general information about macronutrients in their diet but there are countless different opinions, myths, marketing, beliefs, and experiences. Right now let's focus on protein. A war rages on between vegans and meat-eaters about how much protein you need and which sources are the best for the human body. I don't want to engage in a battle but what I will tell you is energy mastery is all about learning to listen to and live in harmony with your body. And your body's needs aren't always the same. I became a vegetarian at age eleven for the intuitive reason that I didn't want to eat meat, but I was a junk food vegetarian eating an abundance of carbs. Over the years I learned to cut down on processed carbs and eat more plants. I also found protein helps me stay full and reduces muscle soreness after working out. I always have a tub of organic fermented vegan protein in the cupboard. You need to get enough variety of amino acids in your diet to form complete proteins. Amino acids are the building blocks of protein and complete proteins are foods containing all nine of the essential amino acids.

Many foods contain some of the amino acids and not others. There was a claim made in the 1980s that you need to get complete proteins together in one meal, however, the author of that information has since retracted her statement, and science has proven as long as you get enough amino acids to form complete proteins within one to two days of each other you will be fine to make the proteins your body needs to be healthy and do all of the amazing processes it does for you every day.

Amino acids are the building blocks of many of your body's cells, tissues, and muscles. There is protein in almost everything, even fruits and vegetables. Just ask the raw-foodists. You can combine celery and cucumber and make a complete, easily digestible protein!

My favorite thing about protein is it keeps you grounded. When you embark on the journey to energy mastery you are lighting up your energy body, embracing your spiritual side, and sometimes getting lost in the possibilities. When you eat protein you become more centered in your heart and mind, feeling calm and dedicated to complete all tasks ahead of you. I'm not going to give you a specific chart or number to aim for as you can find those anywhere online. Notice, when you are feeling anxious or flighty, having some protein can bring you back to your center. If your carbohydrate intake has increased too much and you are feeling bloated or heavy or have other symptoms like brain fog, or fatigue you can increase your protein intake and this should naturally help you reduce your carb intake.

Now more on carbohydrates. Which are the best to ingest and how much is enough or too much? Again it all comes back to knowing your body. You may wish to visit an alternative practitioner such as a Naturopathic Doctor to get some blood and other health tests to dive deeper into the science of your body. For this book, I want to make it clear that fruits and vegetables are carbohydrates. You may not think of them this way as you may think of bread, rice, and pasta as carbs, which they are, but this is a problem when you forget fruits and veggies are carbs too, so you overdo them. Carbs are an important source of energy for your body, especially if you are very active.

Most processed foods are high in carbs and these types of carbohydrates turn into sugar quickly in your body which raises your blood sugar and can leave you with an energy crash or even more cravings after you've eaten. This was a vicious cycle I lived in for years! I was overdoing the carbs and had a daily three in the afternoon crash leaving me wanting a nap and a coffee. It was hurting my work, self-esteem, and on top of it I was so bloated I was asked multiple times when I was due, as in people thought I was pregnant when I was not, I was unhealthy and bloated. How embarrassing!

While gluten is technically a protein, it is often found in carbohydrate-rich products like bread and pasta. Going gluten-free, even if you do not have celiac disease, can have a profound impact on your mood and energy level. If you haven't tried it I highly suggest it! I notice for myself when I overdo gluten for a day or three I feel less energetic and even mildly depressed. Since I have self-awareness (the first key in energy mastery), I can cut all gluten out of my diet and feel incredible again in a day or two after clearing out my system. If I was perfect (and no one is), I would never eat gluten but I'm not celiac and I enjoy some homemade bread and other glutenous treats made with love once in a while.

You'll want to get your carbs from plants, starchy root vegetables, and low glycemic fruit like berries as much as possible. Organic gluten-free grains are also good choices if you are new to making changes or need the carbs for energy. Organic brown rice and quinoa are my faves, and I make a pot to have on hand once every week or two. That way it's ready and when I'm hungry I have a healthy carb choice to throw in salads or stir-frys.

Sugar is a simple carbohydrate, highly refined, and highly addictive. It hides in countless processed and packaged foods because it tastes good and manufacturers know you will buy more if you get hooked on it. Sugar causes your blood sugar to spike which causes a release of the hormone insulin, which then helps your body bring the sugar into the cells lowering the blood sugar. Another glorious act of homeostasis! When you consume too much sugar your cells can become resistant to the effects of insulin, or you lose your ability to produce insulin altogether, this is diabetes which can have all sorts of terrible complications from painful neuropathy (nerve pain) to blindness among other afflictions.

Processed sugar is something you need to take control of in your life. Many people live under its control, reaching for sugary goods after meals to feel satisfied (aka dessert), or needing their afternoon pick me up.

Sugar can make you feel good and give you energy in the short term but in the long term, it will rob your body of energy and nutrients, creating addiction and cycles of undernourishment that are hard to get out of. How do you overcome sugar addiction? Again it starts with awareness. Take an inventory of the foods you are eating and how much sugar is in them, as well as how you feel after eating them. Then with this awareness begin to slowly make better choices. Notice when you need that pick-me-up and choose some protein and a piece of fruit instead of the granola, muffin, or chocolate bar. Eat protein in the morning to put you on solid ground for the rest of your day. And if you find you have a problem with sugar do some journaling around it, why do you like it so much, what feelings does it provide for you? Have you been sold on the idea that eating sweets will make you feel better? Are you missing sweetness in other areas of your life? Recognize that in reality, over the long term, sugar will make you feel worse than if you took excellent care of your health.

Consider when you are craving sweets it may be because there is a lack of sweetness in your day-to-day life, whether it is from outside sources or people, or yourself. When you find yourself craving sweets, offer yourself some sweetness in ways other than food. Buy yourself a small treat such as your favorite magazine or flowers, give yourself a mini massage or go for a full body massage, tell yourself sweet nothings, or request them from your partner or friends. And don't be afraid to go first, offer kind words everywhere you go, and eventually they will ripple back into your world.

An effective way to curb sugar cravings on the spot is to keep a bottle of bitters handy. Bitter is a flavor and there are specific plants that have this quality. The North American diet, which is finding its way around the world, is drastically deficient in bitter flavor. When you embrace bitterness in your palate, your taste buds naturally begin to change to want more balance of other flavors, and less sweetness. You can find a tincture of bitters at any health food store. If you eat more sugar than is good for you regularly I suggest starting with taking the bitters in a bit of water three times a day before meals. This will stimulate your digestion and retrain your taste buds away from sugar. You can also take bitters at any moment when you are having a craving for sweets. The bitter taste will immediately quell the craving and help you reorient towards healthy choices.

I suffered from sugar addiction for many years and know firsthand how it can seem uncontrollable. But I guarantee you if you decide to overcome and follow these simple ideas you can beat it. Ideally, you have no processed or refined sugar in your diet. If that seems too unrealistic in a culture that thrives on sugar and feeding each other sweets on holidays and special occasions (congratulations it's your birthday, lets' feed you some crap!), then start slow. Aim to reduce your sugar, fill your fridge with produce, indulge on special occasions, and fully enjoy it. Know that who you are ultimately is a healthy person who makes the right choices more often than not, and you are working your way up to most of the time. You got this!

If you are into label reading (an excellent habit to have) make it a rule to never buy anything that has more than ten grams of sugar per serving. That is a generous amount, and if you can keep it under five grams you are on the right track. Better yet, don't buy anything in a box that requires labeling. But when you do, read the labels, check for harmful ingredients, and keep the sugar content low.

Now onto the final macronutrient, fat.
Fat has been demonized for years but thankfully you now know better. Fat is an essential part of your diet. What matters is the quantity and quality of fat. In the 1980's fat was deemed as near evil in the media which gave birth to the fat-free foods you now see on grocery shelves everywhere.

But here's the kicker, fat = flavor.

To make all those fat-free foods taste good guess what they did? They added tons of sugar. And what does sugar do in your body, it turns into fat! And on that note, real fat doesn't turn into fat in your body. It can, as can any type of calories when eaten in excess, but the myth that fat makes you fat has no bearing in science any longer.

Fat is crucial for flavor and satiety. It makes your body's hormones happy and it can increase the hormone leptin which suppresses the appetite and makes you feel fuller longer. It can also help decrease the hormone ghrelin, which can make you feel hungry even when you are not.

Healthy fat, in small quantities, is your friend.

Fat is an essential macro-nutrient that gives structure to every single one of your cells! Your tissues and even bones are lubricated with substances made of fat, and your brain is made up of sixty percent fat.

If you are one of those people who are afraid of fat let me tell you politely to get over it already!

Fat is not the enemy.

Now let's talk about quality. Margarine is not good for you in any sense. If you think it is then you have been brainwashed by big marketing. Margarine is one molecule away from being plastic. Your body cannot assimilate it. Margarine is more likely to cause oxidative damage to your tissues, specifically blood vessels, than if you eat real butter and cream on occasion.

High-quality fats are unrefined oils like coconut, olive, grapeseed, sesame, and other UNREFINED nut and seed oils, and avocados. If you enjoy animal products then grass-fed butter, ghee, and animal fats in moderation can add immense flavor and nutrition to your food while making you feel satisfied for longer periods. The take-away energy mastery lesson on fat is to eat fewer refined carbs, focus on produce and healthy fats, and notice how you feel.

Now that we've covered macro-nutrients, fats, carbs, and protein, let's talk about food combining.

Food combining is an incredible principle that teaches you how to eat your food for the best possible digestion. It is simple; combine macronutrients properly, and light to heavy.

Foods that digest easily should be eaten first or on their own such as fruits, greens, and simple carbohydrates. These foods are broken down in under thirty minutes in your stomach. They digest quickly. If you eat these light foods after heavier foods like proteins they would sit on top of the protein and ferment in your digestive system creating bloating and gas, yeast, and bacterial imbalances, and other digestive upset.

The general rule of thumb is to eat your foods light to heavy. Fruits and carbs first, then fats and proteins. They are not hard and fast rules, and again energy mastery is all about listening to your body. Play around with these ideas and see what works for you.

Fruits first and on their own.
Starches combine with other starches and veggies,
Proteins combine with other proteins and veggies.
Nuts, legumes, pair only with veggies.

Keep it simple.

For the health of your digestion, you want to drink fluids away from your meals as they can dilute your stomach acid which is working hard to break your food down for you. If you dilute the potency of your digestive acids it will strain your digestive system. You can sip water if needed at meals but avoid large amounts, keep the big gulps to twenty minutes before a meal or two hours after to give your digestion time to do its job.

Then there is coffee and other caffeinated beverages. Drink these before your meal or two hours after. This is because caffeine can cause your sphincters to open prematurely. Specifically, the sphincters (rings of muscle) at the top and bottom of your stomach that keep it closed from the esophagus and small intestine. This can create heartburn, and/or undigested food flowing into your intestines before they should, which can lead to not only bloating and gas but other digestive problems which may be related to allergies, eczema, and other inflammatory conditions.

Another issue about caffeine is society's dependence on it. Many people drink more than two cups a day. They feel they "need it" to have the energy required to do their jobs. Caffeine is like a false start that can rob your body of its natural energy over time. When you drink caffeine or other caffeinated beverages your adrenal glands get zapped a little when they release adrenaline. Add caffeine to poor sleep patterns, and overall stress in life and you have a disaster waiting to happen for your adrenals leading to burnout and exhaustion. This can be a vicious cycle if you don't listen to your body and continue drinking more caffeine trying to make it through instead of taking a break, lowering your caffeine, and giving your body, mind, and spirit the rest and nourishment it truly needs.

Now I'm not saying you can never have coffee, I am drinking an organic cup 'o' joe as I type this. You do need to be aware that you are not reliant on stimulants and begin to lower your tolerance for them so they can be used as needed or truly enjoyed.

If you are someone who drinks a lot of caffeine I encourage you to begin to cut back. If you drink three cups a day, cut back to two. If you drink two cups a day, cut back to one, if you drink one cup a day cut back to half-caf, and so on. If you have any withdrawal symptoms be sure to hydrate hydrate hydrate!

Hydration helps clean your body out and raise your energy naturally. I'm sure you've heard the phrase "your body is eighty percent water", well caffeine is dehydrating so when you consume it you must drink more water! The general rule of the eight cups a day is potentially adequate if you sit all day and don't exercise at all. And even in this case, most people aren't drinking enough. I like to advise people to drink two to three liters a day minimum. And the quality of water is also important. Your tap water is full of chlorine and other chemicals that destroy the beneficial bacteria in your gut. Also, the structure of tap water isn't easy for the body to absorb. I recommend pure spring water if you can source it. Distilled water is pure and can help with detoxification, and some machines on the market can produce high-quality alkaline water but they can be pricey and you need to make sure they are cleaned regularly so they don't build up with rust or bacteria.

As you increase the amount of water you drink and healthy real whole food in your diet, your energy will increase naturally. I am not currently a raw-foodist but I remember when I was I had so much energy I could hardly contain myself! While that may not be the route you choose, I bet you can drink more water, and add more fruits and veggies to your diet. Do it!

Clean burning fuel = more energy for you = less reliance on stimulants such as caffeine.

You may need to nourish your adrenal glands if you've been reliant on stimulants for a long time. For this, I recommend seeing your local Naturopath or health food store and picking up some adaptogens. Adaptogens are herbs to help nourish and restore the endocrine system, specifically the adrenal glands. They promote homeostasis in the body.

It's no secret we live in a busy world. A world that at times can take a serious toll on your body if you aren't nourishing and nurturing yourself. After a stressful and traumatic event, I had adrenal burnout to the point I was sleeping sixteen hours a day and still never felt rested. The missing key was nourishing my adrenal glands back to health with the class of herbs called adaptogens.

Adaptogens are herbal medicines to help the body adapt to stress and normalize bodily processes. If you are high strung and need to calm down, they can help you relax, and if you are weak and fatigued, they can improve stamina and energy levels.

Adaptogens are my favorite herbal medicine! They are incredibly safe for almost everyone, have been used for thousands and thousands of years, and have helped me and almost everyone I know in some way or another.

A lot of things can cause adrenal insufficiency or burnout, but it all comes down to stress. Constant stress with no rest time, ignoring natural cycles, and not listening to the voice within (intuition) are major contributors. Some symptoms of adrenal insufficiency include constant fatigue, poor muscle recovery after workouts (soreness lasting longer than it should), depression, anxiety, and low blood sugar.

Thanks to mother nature, adaptogens can help. My personal favorite is Ashwagandha. Others include Holy Basil, Siberian Ginseng, Rhodiola, Astragalus, Licorice, Schisandra. (Not an inclusive list.)

Adaptogens help in the following ways:

1. Combat stress by regulating hormones, such as cortisol
2. Increase immunity. (You know how you get sick after a stressful time? This can help!)
3. Increasing strength and endurance (Ashwagandha translates to "Strength of a Stallion")

Adaptogens also boost mood, lower cholesterol, improve sleep quality, and enhance memory and brain function.

As you can see, adaptogens are herbal superstars. If you have been drinking too much coffee check them out to help re-balance your adrenal glands. By eating a clean diet with adequate hydration, fiber, healthy fats and proteins, reducing sugar and processed foods, and adding 500 milligrams once or twice per day of an adaptogen like ashwagandha or holy basil you can reduce stress, improve mood, increase immunity and support the endocrine system.

Your endocrine system is made up of the following organs: hypothalamus, pituitary, thyroid, parathyroid, adrenals, pineal gland, and the reproductive organs (ovaries and testes), as well as the pancreas which does double duty for the digestive and endocrine systems.

These organs are all involved in your hormonal health. Maybe you've heard of hormones but aren't sure what they do other than rage when you are a teenager or going through other significant life changes such as pregnancy, menopause, and andropause. The previously mentioned insulin is a hormone that helps with blood sugar regulation. There is also estrogen and progesterone which are well known for their impact on women's health, and testosterone most notably known as a man's hormone. Both sexes have all hormones, in different amounts, and each person has varying amounts depending on their health status, age, diet, family history, and other factors. We humans are beautifully complex!

When your hormones are in balance you feel like you have harmony in your body and your cycles are natural and relatively easy. The female cycle is usually twenty-eight days, and men can have a daily or weekly cycle of hormone level fluctuation. Energy mastery involves listening to your body, knowing your natural cycle, and having proper expectations based on those cycles. Most women for example have various symptoms leading up to and into the first days of their moon cycle. While this can cramp their style (literally), it's important to listen to the body and give it the rest it needs while it's doing what it is designed to do.

There are various apps and journals you can use to track your cycles and get to know yourself better through your nature. The moon cycle is a sacred time for women as it connects you to your body and the earth. One of my teachers once told me, "It is when the veils between the physical and spiritual are at their thinnest so you have heightened access to divine wisdom, insight, and intuition during this time."

Keeping a journal of how you feel on certain days can help you maximize your radiance when you know what to expect and can plan for it, and give yourself loads of grace when you are not feeling vibrant. Sometimes you need down days to nurture yourself, This is a part of energy mastery. Keeping a journal can help you learn from your mis-takes and keep you going for your goals.

On the topic of vibrancy let's sidestep into alcohol and recreational drugs. In energy mastery, these must be used occasionally at most. When you step into your greatness you will want to feel your best and alcohol and drugs mess up your energy and dull your radiance. Many people rely on drugs and alcohol to get through stressful times or just to let go and have fun. I'm all for stress reduction, letting go, and having fun but the one who has mastered their energy has ways to do this which don't involve harming yourself. If you use these substances or any others that you are aware are interfering with your radiance simply start to cut back. When you feel the urge to indulge notice it and make better choices. Practice letting loose without the substance, or use the substance consciously with intention. I'm a huge proponent of dance parties! Put on your favorite tune and shake your booty, even if for just three minutes. This can help to not take yourself too seriously. You will release stress as you literally shake it off, and it's a great workout. It is also a great tool to help you learn to express your authentic self with innate freedom.

When you are in touch with your authentic self-expression, you must voice your desire to be healthy. First to yourself, then maybe with someone you know will be supportive like a coach or like-minded friend, then to others in your life who may or may not support your lifestyle choices. When other people are involved in your old bad habits, communication is critical. It's important in these times to let other people be themselves while you do you. If they want to overeat or drink and do drugs to drown their sorrows simply let them. If you choose to indulge, be intentional about the use of the substance. Why are you choosing to enjoy it? Is it from escapism or are you adding something to your life or the life of others when you use it?

Breaking old habits and building new ones takes time. Give yourself grace. Know that when breaking an old habit, the best way to do it is to begin starting a new one at the same time. Say you end your day with a glass of wine and it's now second nature. Start to cut back to every second day and on the day you don't drink, drink a liter of water with lemon instead, do some deep breathing, meditate, journal, or go for a brisk walk or run. Break old habits while creating new ones. Be sure to express your needs and desires through your habit-changing process vocally or in writing so nothing gets left behind that can sabotage your success.

Two critical factors in energy mastery that are inseparable are intuition and your gut; ie your "gut feelings". For your gut feelings to be clear and accurate, your gut must be physically healthy. Eating a clean diet can greatly enhance the health of your gut making your gut feelings much clearer. You want to make sure any bacteria and yeast in your digestive system are under control with more healthy bacteria than bad.

Probiotics (you've probably heard of them) are beneficial bacteria living in your gut. When you consume a diet of highly processed and sugary foods, as well as drink alcohol and take pharmaceutical drugs you throw off the balance of good bacteria in your gut which allows bad bacteria, and yeast to thrive. Bad bacteria can cause all sorts of problems from leaky gut, bloating, diarrhea, gas, yeast infections, and even skin disorders such as eczema have their root cause as bacterial dysbiosis (dysbiosis is a term for imbalance, meaning there are more harmful bacteria than good. It is the opposite of homeostasis).

Aside from bacteria and yeast, other creepy creatures that live in your guts are parasites. Parasites are organisms that live on their host and everybody has them. But if your gut is unhealthy you risk having more and letting them grow beyond what is healthy.

Parasitic infections are a real risk factor when traveling to foreign countries. If you've ever traveled and come back with a stomach bug there is a chance you picked up a parasite along the way. Much of the time although you may not feel right, you don't do anything about it, and maybe it goes away or maybe it slumbers in your body, slowly draining you of certain nutrients leading to ill health over time.

Everyone should do a parasite cleanse at least once in their life. Perhaps even every two years if you want to maintain the health of your gut, especially if you travel a lot. Parasite cleanses are combinations of different anti-parasitic herbs like wormwood, black walnut, thyme, cassia, clove, and other ingredients to cleanse the colon.

I remember the first time I did a parasite cleanse. I was skeptical but when I saw a dead parasite in the toilet one day it freaked me out when I realized that sucker had been living on my body for God knows how long. I was glad to get it out!

It is important to do a parasite cleanse over the full moon. Most cleanses last two to three weeks, and you want the middle of it to be when the full moon hits. If you've ever worked in retail or customer service you might have heard "the full moon brings out the crazy in people". Well, this has more to it than the position of the moon, how it affects the water, and horoscopes and such. The eggs parasites lay in your body usually hatch during the full moon. That's enough to bring out the crazy in anyone when you think about possibly hundreds of tiny creatures hatching in your body over a few days. When you do a cleanse over the full moon you have the best chance of wiping most of them out as the herbs will be in your system, there to kill the new hatchlings so they can't latch onto you. I realize this may be gross, disgusting, and even scary information. Sorry about that, the main point is bad bacteria and parasites can drain your energy! Take care of your gut! A clean diet and hydration with pure water are key!

Your gut is also known as your "second brain". Your gut does so much for you and is intertwined with many other systems in the body such as the nervous system and immune system. Also, the endocrine system is connected with the gut. The diet you eat affects the hormones that get produced and the hormones that get produced can move through the digestive system. Think how important your gut is!

In North America, we have been shaming our guts for such a long time. Saying it's too big or too fat. Look at all the pictures of the Buddha, a smiling man with a huge gut! It may or may not be healthy for us to have huge guts, but the point here is to be kind to your belly. Look down right now and tell it you love it, (Seriously do it, and listen to how it reacts).

I used to hate my stomach for years and years as a young woman, and I also didn't know how to listen to it. It seemed bloated all the time. But when I decided to love it, care for it, clean it up, it took on a new role as a trusted advisor, guiding me through my emotions instead of being a place to stuff them. All of my stuffing emotions and eating poorly for the first part of my life and not listening to my gut caused some damage to my body that I have mostly reversed through diet, energy healing, listening, and love, but it takes consistent care now to truly listen. It is a part of my life that helps me, not something to be hated or shamed.

How will you honor your gut and how it guides you in life? Is there a practice you can take on that will help you get more in tune with your gut and how it works for you? In energy mastery, you cannot ignore any part of yourself because you are whole. It takes uncovering all you have stuffed, ignored, shamed, buried, or hidden away and cleaning out the junk, and integrating the lessons of your life. And then opening to all that is beginning to unfold for you. As you clean out the old you make way for more clarity, more mastery, more truth of the love you are. Then you shine forward and be a beacon for others. As you lift yourself (with help as you need it, I take all the help I can get), you permit others to lift themselves, and on and on it goes. Those who are willing to take the lead for those who follow, and eventually those who follow step into their greatness. It's win-win-win all around!

Winning at the health and nutrition game long-term requires diligence and "work" but as you master your energy the "work" becomes a part of who you are and it no longer seems like work, it is who you are. Create the vision of yourself as healthy. Hold the vision, think about it often, deeply connect with it. Create your personal meditation using some background music infused with positive healing tones and your voice stating your goals in the present ie "I am healthy, vibrant, and energetic and I love it!" Make it as long or as short as you like. Listen to it two times a day, let it sink in, become the vision you have for yourself, and own your great ability to make it happen. You got this! Use journals or other apps to stay on track and surround yourself with people who support you and will pick you up when you fall. And when you fall, recognize it, surrender to the experience, and make a choice to move on and begin again. It will get easier over time.

Remember: Eat a mainly whole food, plant-based diet, hydrate hydrate hydrate, and get to know your body so you can tell when you are on track or not and move forward from there, always staying connected to your vision of your healthiest self. If you need support please contact me and we will work on this together.

> **"Let food be thy medicine, and let medicine be thy food."**
> Hippocrates

Health is a total experience. Continually seeking what feels best and implementing actions towards your highest vision, combined with the scientific knowledge of nutrition and bodily processes, will lead you on the path of radiant health.

P.S. Sometimes what feels good in the moment and what is best for us over the long term can seem in conflict. As you deepen your knowledge of self and commit to your own highest good, this conflict can dissipate *as what is truly best for you becomes what feels good now*, in Your Present Moment. You also become comfortable with the uncomfortable as you hold your vision and move through any remaining obstacles to its fulfillment. One of the main obstacles is negative self-talk which we will cover in the next chapter.

Chapter 3

Love Thyself

> Become aware of self-talk.
> This is the first step.
> Become aware.
> Listen.
> What are you saying to yourself?

Jesus said, "...Love your neighbor as yourself." (Matthew 22:39)

Over the years of my journey, as well as working with others I have pondered the question of how good we are doing at this as a society with so much secret self-loathing under the surface of our lives. In my life, I hated myself for so long. While my life was normal and good on the outside, every time I looked in the mirror I judged myself harshly, wondered why I couldn't be prettier, thinner, more attractive, successful, lovable, worthy, etc. This underlying loathing colored my perceptions, interactions with and ability to fully love others. Some people may feel good about the way they look but struggle with self-worth in other ways such as intelligence, humor, or likeability.

My self-hatred made me vulnerable to narcissists who would only lift me up to drag me down. After getting out of a particular instance of falling prey to one of these narcissists and dedicating my life to truth and healing, I discovered that I had no idea who I truly am! I had a vague sense I wanted to be a good person and live a good life, but I wasn't connected with my heart, voice, or power. I didn't honestly love myself the way I deserve. Through seeking mentors who could help me uncover my shadows and past experiences that created this web of self-loathing around me I uncovered my voice, and let go of the past patterns of self-sacrifice and unkindness to self. Through this, I deepened my ability to love others and I learned to love all of me, even during the messy, complicated times.

Self-love begins within and the best place to start is by watching your self-talk. As we learn to fully love ourselves, we can truly love others even more. Many people are incredibly harsh on themselves inside their mind and this chapter will help you release this habit for good.

If you don't get a handle on your negative self-talk there is no room to expand into greatness. The negative voices will take you out time and time again as you try to rise. The negative thoughts are sticky and take a lot of work to get unstuck. But the work is worth it! You must be firm but gentle with yourself, and hard on the lies. Kick the good-for-nothing, useless, life-sucking lies out!

As you gain awareness of how you talk to yourself, you can begin to witness it without judgment and simply inquire where it is coming from. You might ask "whose voice is it anyway?" You may have taken on the voices of your parents or partners, and when you are aware of this you can change that so you listen to the truth of love whispering within.

Sometimes it can be hard to separate who you are from your self-talk and this is why meditation is such a wonderful practice. You must start to listen. You are listening for your inner guidance, but if you're like most, including me, you have to get through all the nonsense thoughts before you can get clarity. With practice and time, it gets easier.

Self-talk can be tricky. Sometimes as your heart and soul get stronger your ego also gets stronger. You must remain diligent and treat yourself and others with love at all times. You must practice this and begin to take control. A tip I learned is to wear an elastic band around your wrist and whenever you notice a negative thought snap it and say "thank you for sharing". This acknowledges the thought without giving it any energy and "snaps" you back to the truth, which is that you are enough.

I wonder if you will try this for even a week? Go on, I dare ya! And then let me know how it goes.

Until you can master your negative thoughts, the ones that seemingly come out of nowhere, so they are few and far between, it's a great idea to begin choosing and reciting positive thoughts. Now, this can be tricky since you don't want to start saying things to yourself you don't inherently believe are true. You wouldn't go around affirming "I am happy and fulfilled" if you are depressed and feel stuck in your life. This is a recipe for disaster where your ego can talk back to you with things like "yeah right, that's not true". You want to use affirmations about the qualities you are striving to embody. For example. "I am strong enough to create what I want" is a good one.

The same goes for money thoughts. There are a lot of gurus out there who tell you to recite grandiose affirmations every day such as "I am a billionaire!" and there's nothing wrong with that except if your inner-self talks back. Mine always did when I started using affirmations in my late twenties. I used big grand affirmations and my inner self was always responding with "no, you're not!" It was like trying to put fancy words over old wounds and ingrained beliefs without actually healing them. As I realized this, I began shifting what I was saying to more embodiment words and phrases such as "I am enough" and "I am smart and can create what I truly desire in my life" and "I am discerning what I truly want and will create from there" and "I am creating x amount of dollars in these types of accounts, and using my money this way for the highest and best good of all". This felt way more empowering for me and I've generated massive results since using these types of phrases. Try one on for yourself. I'm particularly fond of "I am enough" as most limiting beliefs are rooted in "not-enoughness".

I have a love/unlove relationship with affirmations and here's why. Most of us who have learned about the law of attraction and the use of affirmations in our lives have learned about them from a place of lack, or being or having "not enough". We then take on this practice from that place. It's hard to feel one hundred percent congruent when you are reciting words out loud which deep down you don't believe.

How can you truly embody your affirmations? It starts again with awareness and daily practice. Be aware first of your thoughts, and then how you feel when you hear your thoughts, as well as how you truly feel when you are stating your affirmations. For example, if you are saying "I am a millionaire" but your inner child is screaming "no I'm not, there's not enough!" and the voice of a parent or another person is in your head saying "money doesn't fall out of the sky you know dear" then there is some deeper work to be done than just the reciting of affirmations.

We will dive deeper into this in the chapters to come but for now, be aware of the thoughts and feelings arising as you begin taking on more positive self-talk and embodiment-based affirmations. As you are creating your affirmations you want them to truly come from the heart. Listen to your heart for what it wants to express. Use empowering language. If you don't believe something such as "I am a millionaire" use words such as "I am becoming a person who can earn, grow, and keep larger sums of money".

The lesson is, if it doesn't feel right, there is no point in trying to force it. Listen to your true feelings and use your journal to help uproot them. Better yet, reach out to a qualified coach or healer such as myself to help you get to the root and release it once and for all and find what is true for you. I use money affirmations as an example because it seems like the world got swept away with the Law of Attraction and focused a lot on the material world. There is nothing wrong with that but when you are looking at images of things and bumping up against the old beliefs saying you lack those things then you may create more lack.

Isn't it interesting that two years after the movie The Secret came out there was the 2008 financial crisis and housing market crash? Isn't it funny there was a hit movie that taught about the law of attraction and vision boards, and shortly thereafter millions lost their homes and the stock market crashed harder than it had since the great depression in 1929?

This is important to ponder as you potentially make your vision board as well. I have had a difficult time creating vision boards using magazine cut-outs in the past because the images I found didn't resonate and didn't reflect what I truly wanted. With some guidance from a great intuitive coach, I was encouraged to hand draw my vision board. What I created was exactly what I wanted and after putting the vision board on my wall I fell in love more and more with my path to manifesting my vision every day.

Do you have a vision board? If so, take a minute and ponder if it is truly reflective of your heart's desires. And if you don't have one, take the time to create one. Magazine cut-outs are ok, *just make sure whatever you create is an external representation of what is on the inside trying to manifest through you, not a representation of some external thing you are trying to get.*

You can come up with some incredibly personalized affirmations through this reflective process. Instead of reciting words with little meaning, feel into the energy of your vision and create your affirmations from there. This will be how you truly embody your truth and begin to expand from the inside out.

You may notice as you do this work that old beliefs, patterns, and traumas may rear their heads. This happens because you truly evolve from the inside out. When you are expanding yourself from your heart anything living in the body, energetically or physically, will get pushed up and out. This is the process of energetic transformation and why awareness of yourself is so important. As you begin to embody your truth you may need to work with another to address the fears that arise, old memories that come up, or anything else blocking you from your continued success. If you feel stuck never hesitate to ask for help. Asking for help, even though it puts you in a vulnerable state, is a powerful thing to do! No one successful would be where they are today without help.

Keep at it, one day at a time you become new, embodying your truth and releasing the past. Over time it becomes easier as you become stronger in your authentic self. Permit yourself to be amazing. As you claim your unique authority in your own life, beginning with the thoughts in your mind you can begin to make more deliberate choices. By not looking outside for permission to be great and do what you want, you empower yourself to be all you can be.

You may have old imprints from what you previously believed is acceptable. These imprints and beliefs can be completely subconscious until brought to light through conscious inquiry. When analyzed you can see how these imprints are holding you back. When you analyze where they came from and apply them in your current context you can see how crazy it is to have the same set of rules you learned to follow as a child governing your life as an adult!

As you set new rules and ways of being you can create a new identity based on your core values. You can create a new identity, based on the truth, that you are connected to Divine all-powerful love.

Take out your journal now and write at the top:

"Your name's Identity" (ie. Anne Smith's Identity)

Then write out words describing who you truly are and who you want to be. You can even ask your friends and family how they would describe you.

Then on another page write:

"Who is Your name". (ie Who is Anne Smith)

Write out who you are for three to five minutes in sentence form.

Finally, on a new page write:

"Character traits of your name". (ie Character traits of Anne Smith)

Write ten to twenty words such as caring, kind, honest, punctual, and when you are done write a small phrase about how you embody those traits next to each word.

Once you have done this, review it daily for a week. I also recommend creating your very own personalized meditation using these pages. I put some soft music on my laptop, then using my smartphone I record myself speaking the phrases and words over the music. I repeat it until I have created a five to fifteen-minute meditation. Then listen to this once or twice a day, it will start to get in your head and push out the negative thoughts as your subconscious absorbs these new truths.

Imagine the impact of waking up each day with these truths going into your mind, and falling asleep each night with a reminder of who you truly are!

Over time you want to own this new identity from spirit, not ego. You can do this by continually returning to your heart. Here is a simple exercise to get you there.

Visualize a golden ball of light in the center of your head.

Begin counting backward from ten to one, bringing the golden ball of light lower with each count and landing in your heart at number one.

Once the ball of light lands in your heart, breathe deeply into your heart in the center of your chest and see your heart opening.

Open it on the front. Breathe.

Open the back of the heart. Breathe.

Open the left and the right sides of the heart. Breathe.

Open the top and the bottom of the heart. Breathe.

Breathe deeply for a few breaths allowing your heart to expand in all directions and open even more.

Feel how that feels.

Get comfortable with this energy and allow the energy of your heart to move through your whole body. Down your arms and into your torso and legs, and up your neck into your mind.

Take a few breaths and allow this energy to settle within you.

This exercise strengthens the heart and allows you to lead a heart-led life. By strengthening the heart you can begin putting your ego-mind in service to your heart instead of letting the ego-mind control you. Use this exercise to claim your new identity for good. After dropping into your heart is a great time to listen to your heart, and speak its truths. Overcoming negative self-talk and living from your new identity takes diligent awareness but I guarantee if you take this practice on it will be a pleasure to implement and not just another thing on the to-do list.

After you've done this exercise for the first time you may want to journal. And speaking of journals, on the journey to energy mastery you can think of your journal as your new therapist. Use your journal to reflect on your day, free flow your thoughts, remind yourself of your goals, and get your frustrations out through the pen. I have been journaling for years. My first book, *Connect, Strengthen, Surrender*, which is available online in e-book format, was created from writings in my journals.

Journals are also amazing because over time you can look back and see how far you've come. How many goals have you reached and realizations about your truth have you embodied?

If this is a difficult question to answer it's ok. Life is a never-ending journey of personal evolution and creation. You can use all feedback you receive, both from others and through your internal self, to guide the way forward.

~Breakthrough on Demand~

One of the most powerful ways to use your journal is to create breakthroughs on demand. If you have committed to doing something but you "just don't feel like it", or other legitimate or illegitimate reasons/excuses why you can't do it try this; sit with your journal and write something like "I told myself I would…" and continue. Write out how you feel about it now, what's getting in the way, and why you don't want to do it. As you write these things out you will see how those thoughts are energy and as you write them out they lose power. Once you have completed writing all you can you will find you have created the space and energy to do the thing. Next time you feel stuck give it a try. While this seems simple it is truly life-changing.

~Say Goodbye to Your old Self~

It can be therapeutic to say goodbye to your old self. Like skin cells regenerating from the lower levels of your dermis, you are also regenerating from the inside out. Think about it, you know inherently your true light shines from within, this is the source of your power.

As you step into your new core identity, you may want to hold a ceremony for your old or younger self, the one who has been through all the trials and tribulations of life thus far. This may look like writing yourself a letter thanking yourself for all you have grown through. Or it might look like an Epsom salt bath where you visualize the hot water soaking all of the old out of you and letting it wash down the drain while you emerge from the tub refreshed and renewed.

Ceremonies are a potent way to mark beginnings and endings. In western culture, it is often marked by baptisms, weddings, and funerals. But there is much more. Holding a ceremony is a way to bring the sacred into life as it is needed, which may not necessarily line up with life's so-called biggest events.

With any ceremony, you want to have clear intentions going in. In the example above; the desire to release your old self with love and gratitude, a ceremony is a process of honoring all that has been and welcoming in the new. This is not a time to hurry or want things to be different. But a time to truly let go and live on.

By strengthening your heart and inner light and letting go of the old you step into your greatness. Letting go of the past is a continual process once you have learned to master your energy and healed the things in your life that were weighing you down and holding you back. Things are constantly coming up, circumstances happen, relationships change, jobs change, challenges come up. You want to learn to embrace all of these experiences with love and let them go as gently as you can. It's ok to struggle with this as well, remain aware, self-care the heck out of yourself, and be willing to constantly let go (without bypassing your true feelings about situations) and uplevel into your truth. Meditation is crucial for this awareness.

Learning to quiet my mind and listen to my thoughts has been profound in my own life. As I have uprooted and uncovered old limiting beliefs and perceptions about myself I have replaced them with mightier truths that put me on the path to energy mastery which I now teach others. Simply sitting and listening is an easy first step to awareness and when implemented can have a massive impact on your life, which you can then use to help others.

Once you have become aware of your self-talk you will start to notice the things other people say that are disempowering about themselves or others. You can lovingly point this out to help lift everyone up. While writing this chapter I heard a friend of a friend emasculate himself harshly at an event. Though he said it with humor I pointed out that your words have power and you should do your best to only say positive things about yourself. When you let people know where they can gain awareness and better their lives they are almost always thankful. Some people may get testy or triggered and say it's none of your business, in that case, let it be. They may have an aha moment later and even though they seemed put off you may have helped them make a major turning point in their life. If they don't receive any insight, it's none of your business. Don't take their reaction personally.

We've all met people who are physically beautiful but have buried their light so far inside themselves it's hard to see. Don't worry about them, focus on shining your light.

Side note on worry > Worry is wasted. Wasted time and energy. If you notice yourself worrying, take a pause, call your whole self in and make a different choice. Talk to the person or thing you are worried about, pray for a positive outcome, journal those worries out, and let them go. Choose happy thoughts, choose gratitude, choose acceptance, and unconditional love for each individual's journey. Worry lives in the ego. Stay in your own heart.

The heart is the center of all transformation but most of society lives in their minds which have become stronger than the heart. To access the heart, you must quiet the mind and learn to reprogram the mind for openness and service to the heart. Your conscious and subconscious mind is like the captain and crew of your life. The heart is the wide ocean or vastness of space holding it all.

The conscious mind is like the captain. It tells your subconscious mind, the crew, what to do. From about age seven, you can make up your mind and direct yourself. This is why having awareness of and making a conscious effort to think positive thoughts is critically important.

Your subconscious mind, the crew, takes information from the conscious mind and programs paradigms and concepts into the fabric of your being. These programs essentially run your life so you want to make sure they are good!

We have talked about becoming aware of the programs and patterns, now it is time to start creating and implementing new ones. You may have heard of this as "reprogramming your mind". Here are some tips to do this effectively to produce the results you desire. To reprogram your mind takes two core ingredients; repetition and emotion! You must repeat the new programs, ideas, and concepts over and over and over again. You are rewriting your way of being. But you can't just say it over and over in monotone, you must add emotion and feeling and passion behind the words. Don't only repeat the words "I am healthy" over and over but stand up, walk fast while stating emphatically "I am creating impeccable health! I deserve to feel my best and I want to be my best!!!" and then clap your hands and snap your fingers to help it truly settle into the subconscious. Even better is if you do this while remembering a time in your life when you did feel amazing. In Neuro-Linguistic Programming, this is called "anchoring".

If you do this enough (repeat!) you can create a trigger for positive feelings in life. You may think of triggers as "I'm triggered" in a bad way. For example, someone said something that reminded you of something and causes you to want to self-sabotage or get angry or withdraw. These are triggers, which can be unraveled, but here you are focused on creating your positive triggers. When you've made your emphatic statement and clapped your hands and snapped your fingers while feeling amazing you are anchoring this state into your being. Then, when you are feeling low and have been lazy or are reaching for the ice cream or anything that isn't in alignment with your best self, you can clap your hands and snap your fingers which will create a cascade of positive energy and emotion in your body to interrupt the behaviors you no longer want.

Reprogramming your mind and essentially your way of being is like rinse and repeat on overdrive. You must stay focused on where you are going, why you want it, and do the work to get there. I'm all for the law of attraction but it doesn't mean you can sit in your room and meditate all day thinking all that you want will come to you. Meditating is helpful and it will draw things to you but you must become the kind of person who already has those things! Creation is an action word so go for it. Stay open to all the amazing possibilities, and enjoy the ride!

The more you pay attention to your thoughts, be kind and loving to yourself, and start to claim your power through reprogramming your mind, the more you create space for your true self, your heart, to emerge. It's important to be diligent with this. If you find negative thoughts and old, unsupportive ways of being creep back in, as they are likely to, notice and take new action. Rinse and Repeat! And if you find things from your past are coming up and getting in the way and you can't break through them please reach out. Ask for help. I've got space and time to help you. You don't have to go it alone. Call in all the support you can handle and grow as far as you can in this life. Reach for your full potential. You've got nothing to lose and that which you fear you might lose is most likely what you no longer want or need anymore anyway.

Watching your thoughts and claiming your sovereignty over your mind is ultimately up to you. Begin within, then reach out for help along the way. Take full responsibility for your life and watch your divine path unfold with a love you never imagined possible! Now that you've mastered your self talk it's time to listen deeply to your heart and soul. Keep reading to learn how to connect with and follow your heart and intuitive guidance.

Chapter 4

Follow Thy Heart

What does "follow your heart" mean anyway?

As much as you try, you can't escape it. The still small voice is getting louder. For the past few centuries, this inner voice has been ignored, beaten down, and trampled on in the name of "progress" and materialism. In the current age, this voice, which comes from inside, is calling more and more people to awaken to their divine gifts and use them for the new beneficial progress and spiritual evolution of mankind.

Still many people today (myself included), spend their formative years ignoring this voice. Or in my case, completely forgetting it is there. We grow up and march on to do all the things society calls us to do, which are not necessarily bad, but we do them with such drive we forget to slow down and listen to the truth that whispers within. Eventually, the truth needs to be heard. Many people find themselves in crises for having not listened to the voice of the divine. The divine won't put up with it anymore and in due time calls people to their true greatness. This process can be painful for some, as they learn to let go of all they held dear as true. They let go of what society may think about their calling, uncover all of the limited and frankly untrue beliefs they carried their entire lives, and open to the newness they are becoming.

At times during my spiritual awakening and learning to listen to my heart. I felt angry that I was not taught this way of living, I also felt disconnected from many of my friends and family as I became very energetically and spiritually sensitive. As I grew, I had to go through some hard times in my relationships and career. I remember being so sensitive to others' energy as I uncovered my gifts of seeing and feeling that I kept to myself a lot. I later realized my coworkers thought I was a bitch! But actually, I was growing through so much I didn't have any bandwidth left to deal with more people in a day. Over time I grew into my power and now have no problems interacting with a hundred people in a day, but it took time and dedication to become my best and follow my heart even through the tough points. And I wouldn't have it any other way.

If you are on the journey of following your heart and you feel misunderstood, please recognize that this may be an old pattern. Who you truly are is wholly relatable and lovable and capable of loving beyond any differences, for at the core we are all one. If you feel stuck you know you can reach out for help. This is a special time for humanity as we are all called to our divinity. You can't escape this process. Some will try to ignore it or suppress it, but not you or else you wouldn't be reading this book! In moments of doubt know it is love that calls you forward. This love is the core truth of energy mastery. This love is all-powerful, flows from within, and you are never disconnected from it (even when you feel disconnected, ignore it or forget about it)!

When it comes down to it, energy mastery and intuition are all about trusting yourself. Trusting yourself is something many lose over the early parts of life as we learn to listen to outside authority figures instead of ourselves. If you want to truly master your energy you must do the work to trust yourself deeply and all of the information in this book will help you with this. It starts with the desire and intention to truly trust yourself, then by listening to the mental chatter running through your mind and finding your inner truth through meditation.

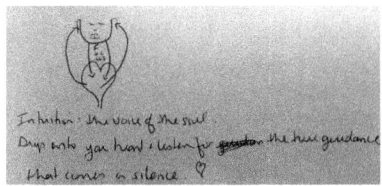

Trusting yourself is about trusting the first answers you receive intuitively. However, most people get answers to their internal questions but then second-guess that answer and keep searching and wondering why they aren't taking action or getting results. They end up acting on the second, third, fourth, or a later thought instead of the original answer. Then they don't get the result they would have gotten had they taken action based on the original guidance. Acting on first intuition is the essence of faith.

It can be hard to start listening to internal guidance when you haven't done it for a while. You can begin by listening to the small nudges you feel, tuning into your gut feelings about people, things, and situations. Even listening to and acknowledging the guidance you are receiving, even if you choose not to act on it now is a step towards greater self-trust. These practices will strengthen your ability to both hear and act on your guidance which over time builds trust in your true self and the Divine who will never lead you astray on your path in life.

Daily quiet time is essential when you are first looking to increase trust in yourself. It stops all the outside influences on your mind and allows you to hear what's going on inside your head and heart. You can then choose to listen to the voice of your heart and soul instead of your ego-mind or outside influences. Begin today, set aside 5 minutes of quiet time, examine your mental chatter, and begin to ask for guidance. If you are comfortable praying, use a simple prayer such as:

"Dear Divine, please show me how to strengthen my trust in my true self and to act according to its guidance. Thank you."

Prayer has a way of cutting straight through any mental B.S. If you don't resonate with the term prayer, simply replace it with "asking" or "intending". You are directing the conversation from your heart-felt intention, and it places you in a state of humble receptivity so the Divine can speak to you.

Choosing to hone intuition is one of the most influential and life-changing decisions you can make. Being deeply connected to and trusting your intuition is a delightful way of being. Begin inquiring of your heart, asking it to guide you today, and see how things open up.

We all receive and experience our connection and guidance in ways that are unique to us. There are many senses with which you can get guidance. Your five physical senses, and the six intuitive senses of "seeing, feeling, hearing, tasting, and smelling", as well as simply "knowing".

There are many ways to discover your intuitive senses and it starts with the curiosity to know more about yourself. I have and experience all of the intuitive senses, with smell being the least present in my experience. Being in tune with yourself means more alignment in your life. As you open to your intuition, the whispers of the Divine become clearer, no matter what channel or sense they come through.

Following your heart is not about the organ of the heart, or the heart chakra, or even just pure intuition. It's a combination of many factors that occur when you are in congruence with your true self and the call upon your life. Embracing the action steps you are guided to take from within will help create the life the Divine has for you, through you. The Great Divine is always listening and guiding. Are you open to it? Your personal evolution occurs in a positive direction when the power and love of divinity flow through you.

Learning to listen to your heart can be incredibly exciting. I remember when I first opened my heart and started listening to it it took me on an epic journey of growth and expansion. I met all kinds of new people, started taking courses to take my learning to new levels, and I felt wonderful. There was one little problem though. I hadn't yet made friends with my mind and pretty much left it out of the picture. This caused some hardship as I hadn't taken care of my finances and made some silly mistakes that took time and effort to remedy. Nothing majorly terrible happened but now I see the wisdom in the phrase:

"Follow your heart but take your brain with you."

Aldred Adler

Your heart should be the center of your life, for, in essence, it is You, expanding and expressing. Your mind is clever and intelligent. Most people's minds are way stronger than their hearts and this can lead them to feel disconnected from themselves. Your mind should be used for practical matters, such as money management, scheduling, and organization. Thinking is crucial to modern life. In energy mastery you make the mind serve the heart. This takes awareness and practice and starts with simply commanding your mind to serve your heart. You can do this now.

Close your eyes and drop into your heart. Visualize surrendering your mind to your heart, envelope your head in the energy of your heart. Breathing deeply into the heart, make it known to the mind that the heart has the reigns. (The heart reigns!) You may need to do this several times. I need reminders from time to time, especially when big opportunities come up. I always listen to my heart first and give my mind the freedom to think it through and share its solutions. This is also where journaling comes in handy. If your mind is losing it, give it a voice through writing and see how quickly the chaos, confusion, and fears of the mind dissipate.

The mind can be tricky but your heart will get stronger, which will impact all areas of your life as your resonance becomes aligned with love and truth. You will develop more faith in yourself as you begin to live from within.

Here is a potent practice to increase your faith in and connection to your true self:

First off start claiming and owning your faith as if you are a king or queen. Make bold declarations about your worth, your value, your beliefs. Call in your faith and ask the Divine for help with this. Do this deliberately, out loud, for as many days in a row as you can. You may remember in a previous chapter I said that when your mind doesn't believe what you are affirming it can talk back. This is not the time to even think of allowing this sort of backtalk. This is you, speaking from your heart, your truth, calling all of you in with love! If something comes up that needs attention, allow it to unravel and learn from it. Use each step to build the faith you are growing in yourself.

As you begin to own your faith and trust your inner guidance, pay attention to self-sabotage, where the lizard brain, the primal part of you focused on basic survival, creeps in and makes you think you don't want the things you do! Know that the lizard brain isn't the real you, it's an old survival mechanism that has greatly served you, and humanity as a whole, but you are now ready to outgrow and overcome. Continually realign with the real you. The real you is pure love, pure power, and pure divinity. This is you! Own it, use it for good. Go ahead, believe it!

As an adult, we sometimes need training in trusting our hearts and intuition. Many of us have self-trust and intuition trained out of us by society as we focus more outward and want to fit in. Even though you sometimes forget about your intuition, which can lead to not trusting it fully, it is always there, your constant companion. Your intuition is kind of like a dog, it's always there, ready to serve and play even after you've ignored it. Intuition is a constant companion offering you a joyful connection to your inner wisdom.

Your intuition is a guide, it may not have all the concrete answers you wish for in difficult times, but it will help you forward one step at a time. Perhaps you've had an experience where you felt out of touch with your intuition for some time and then you had an emergency or crisis and your intuition showed up in full force guiding you through the glaring situation.

When I was in my twenties I wound up in a cult-like situation because I was disconnected from my intuition. I fell prey to ego tricks of the mind but when it got so bad that I needed a way out, I asked for guidance from a higher power I wasn't even sure I believed in, and my intuition took over my whole body and even my environment. One day during that time, I was hurting so badly inside and felt I had nowhere to turn. I locked myself in a bedroom and asked God for an answer about what to do. Instantly and out of "nowhere" I heard and felt and knew my answer. It felt intensely profound, both from within and outside of myself, I knew it was the truth.

Piercing the darkness I found myself in came the light of the words "Get out!". What I heard was simple, as intuition usually is. It didn't console me or coddle me, or even tell me the full details of how to extract myself from my terrible situation. But I knew what I had to do and slowly but surely I began removing my minor possessions from where I lived. Then I built up the courage to tell the man to whom I had been giving my power; "I am leaving."

Even though I had my answer, it wasn't easy.

He threatened me, turned others against me, and made fun of me.

None of that mattered now because I knew what it felt like to have an answer come from within. The clarity and conviction were incredible and something I will never forget. Now, many years later, I know I can access my intuition in all moments, not just moments of crisis.

Here are essential tools for hearing your intuition:

-Daily quiet time. This doesn't necessarily mean meditation but it can if that helps you. Simply BEing in a quiet space will help you reconnect with yourself at the deepest level. Silence is Golden.

-Body scan. Take a few deep breaths and use your mind's eye and all of your senses to scan in and around your body. Notice if there are any areas of tightness or fatigue. You can begin to breathe into those areas or even ask them for a message. If you notice any areas that are light and feel good see if you can expand that energy throughout the rest of your body. The point here is simply to notice the body and invite more lightness into it. The body is your vehicle for life and if you are out of touch with it it's like driving a car blind.

-Cleansing your intuition. Intuition often comes through the center of your head. It is the place of vision. Most people live their lives from their busy ego-mind, therefore intuition is often congested with all the thoughts of the world. To cleanse the intuition simply imagine a white light surrounding your head, washing away all of the negative thoughts and blind spots, and anything that gets in the way of your ability to truly see and perceive. This can be for as little as thirty seconds, up to thirty minutes. The longer you do this, the more heightened your visual sense will be. Begin where you are and do what you can. Be sure to notice the difference before and after in all areas of life.

If you really want to ignite your intuitive abilities, set a timer for five to ten minutes and visualize light coming in from all directions into your intuition and mind for seven days in a row! Be sure to drink lots of water when you do this and if you experience headaches try to avoid taking any painkillers as this pain is a reflection of the cleansing and opening of the energy within.

-Pray for guidance. This doesn't have to take long. A simple prayer in the morning asking your intuition to show up and point you in the right direction can guide you all day long if you keep your mind and heart open to the results. This is not asking for stuff or for things to go your way, but rather to be shown the way. Prayer is most powerful when asking for guidance and to be a vessel of divine service for the highest good of all.

-Finally, listen for your intuition in whatever way resonates most with you, and act on it. It's nice to hear your intuition. It's even nicer to follow it up with action! If you hear it and don't act you can get a backlog of fabulous information that stays with you. When you act on what you hear you often get miraculous results. You are allowing intuition to flow in your life so you get even more intuitive guidance. It's building faith. Listen, act, listen, act, listen, act, and on and on it goes.

Now that you have some tools for hearing your intuition you might be wondering what exactly to use it for in this grand adventure called life. You can use intuition for the tiniest of life situations, to the overall bigger picture. In daily life, it is all about honoring your path. Listen to your intuition for what foods to eat, how to move your body, which people to spend time with. In the bigger picture the small things add up over time, and you begin to take bigger steps. Perhaps the intuition calls you to leave a job or a relationship, go into a certain place, do a specific thing, take a step in one direction, say the words you've been wanting to say. All of these things are you taking steps in the direction of the expression of yourself as love in the world. The world needs more love expressed! And it begins from within, taking the small steps, making the big leaps, all because you have faith and trust in yourself and the Divine.

The best way to get started if you are feeling overwhelmed by all of this, or unsure of how to move forward, or even if you are excited to get started, is to always begin by clearing your energy. This can be as simple as taking a few deep breaths and visualizing a golden waterfall of light pouring down through the top of your head into your body and down into the earth.

When you are using your intuition to help you make a decision you always want to check in, do the ten to one head-to-heart countdown to make sure you are in your heart center. Ask yourself what a "Yes" and what a "No" feels like. Most of the time a "Yes" will feel light, and a "No" will feel heavy. You always want to expand in the direction of lightness. It is important not to ignore the heavy feelings and emotions that sometimes show up. This is the work, unraveling all of the old energy so you can become new. Releasing the old and letting in fresh energy.

When it comes to following your intuitive guidance you might feel hesitant at some of the guidance you receive. I still do sometimes. Only great masters have been able to completely surrender to the divine will. I strive to be one of them but I still have much work to do. The idea is to stretch yourself. Stretch yourself by taking small steps in the direction your intuition is guiding you. Stretch yourself but don't break yourself. One step at a time is often enough. Personal transformation is work and can take time. Don't be discouraged if you don't see results right away or stop because your transformation takes longer than others. You are worth it.

Even though I'm harping on one small action step at a time, it's still critical. You MUST take action! When I first learned about the law of attraction I thought I could meditate and think about external things I wanted and they would magically appear. What a fool I was! The Law of Attraction is all about who you Be. And who you Be, leads to what you Do, and what you do leads to the manifestations of your results.

The law of attraction only works when you do. You might have some luck manifesting things using pure mind strength, yet the divine often gives you what you need and not what you want. Wanting, if not looked into, can often be a state of lack. To want is to not have. To not have is to not Be, according to the Law of Attraction. You must become the vision you have for yourself and the action is where the true transformation occurs. If you are asking yourself for intuitive guidance but not following it up with action, you create a bottleneck of energy which can lead to upset and frustration! Use your power for good and create what you came here to create. Listen to your intuition, and take it one step at a time, always enjoying the journey!

When you truly believe in yourself you **know** one thousand percent that God lives within and is partnered with you. In reality, there is no separation. Beings have consciousness and all consciousness is evolving towards lightness (in the grand scheme of things). When you believe in yourself you don't accept anything other than positive self-talk, there is no room for self-bashing or putting yourself down. No room, zero tolerance, only love. And if you slip up you quickly admit it, atone/apologize, and make a better choice. Out of love for yourself you respect yourself and take full responsibility for your life.

I have known several people from my past who believed in much of the spiritual and energetic principles you are reading about in this book, but they wouldn't apply it in their lives. They loved reading about the theories and talking about them with others, but they never truly integrated the great lessons. These people would go to psychics almost weekly to have their fortune told and they seemed to be addicted to the psychics for their next kick in life. Always wondering if they were going to come into some money or meet a special man, but never taking responsibility, never learning to trust their intuition while giving their power and money away to someone happy to take it. This isn't meant as a dig to psychics, some have a real gift, but you must be careful where so-called psychics get their insights and whether they are using them to honestly empower you or take from you. When you have faith and intuition you can be your own guide. Use your discernment, own your power.

When you own your power you can combine your intuition and your heart to let the Divine guide you on the most amazing journey- the walk of faith which illuminates consciousness and creates real beauty in the world. With your intuition and heart working together it is a divine connection. Your soul, which radiates through your heart, knows the way and you must let the Divine guide you. When you ignore your heart and intuition you create energy stagnancy in your being that weighs you down and holds you back.

A lot of the time I am working with others who are newly stepping into their power, they carry the weight of past regrets and experience, and working together we clear these old energies out so they can live from a place of divine connection and ultimate freedom. Today and every day, invite your heart and the Divine to guide you. When you wake up, first ask your heart how it is doing, tell it you love it, ask it to show you the truth, and invite it to guide you more and more.

Some things that might create blocks to intuition are:

-Sickness; this goes for colds, up to other more serious or critical illnesses. You know the feeling when you have a bad cold. You can't think straight, it's hard to get up and do anything. This is not the time to think too much about following your heart and intuition. Let yourself rest, it's likely what your body needs. Make sure you are hydrated and well-nourished. Perhaps take some immune-boosting vitamins and herbs such as vitamin c and b-vitamins, as well as echinacea, and medicinal mushrooms like reishi and chaga.

Other more serious illnesses which cause pain and suffering can make it difficult to hear your heart and mind, but based on the latest science and millennia of spiritual teachings we know that the body sends us messages when it is out of alignment. If you are suffering from an ailment, seek out as much information as you can and begin listening to your body for guidance on how to heal and live your best life regardless of any physical healing outcome. Make sure you are hydrated, exercise in any way you can, and work with a Naturopathic Doctor, western medicine, and/or any other practitioner you feel comfortable with. I mention Naturopaths specifically as they are skilled at finding and working with root causes in a way that works on its own or in conjunction with western medicine if that is a part of your plan. Chiropractors, acupuncturists, ayurvedic practitioners, nutritionists, massage therapists, and all kinds of alternative modalities can be of assistance in your journey. Ask your heart what resonates with you and go in that direction.

-Trauma locks; when you experience trauma in your life you often hold your breath. As you hold your breath you are holding energy from flowing and when you do this in conjunction with an event that is traumatizing (which can be many things), you create a "lock" in your energy field. The place where the energy can't flow becomes trapped in time and space, impeding further energy flow. Not always entirely but enough to cloud your vision and hold you in fear to some extent. Western society tends to hold onto these things and cover them over with daily life and outer circumstances, medication, or even spiritual bypassing where they pretend everything is ok. As you do the work in this book and expand your heart and consciousness you may uproot some of these trauma locks. As they are released be sure to breathe, allow yourself to feel, and release all of the emotion associated with it. It's just energy (energy in motion= emotion). Emotional releases can manifest as tears, laughter, feeling cold or hot, needing to scream or move the body vigorously. Be aware and let the energy flow in whatever way it comes out.

-Lack of belief; This doesn't need much explanation but to reiterate, if you don't believe in intuition, you are likely to have a hard time listening to and following it. If you were trained to listen to outside authorities over your inner voice you may struggle between the two. Truthfully, if you have good outside advice it most likely won't be at odds with your intuition. A good mentor should help you cultivate your intuition and be a good role model, by living life in congruence with their heart.

-Short-term desires and other outer influences. You know the feeling of the discrepancy between your intuition guiding you to your highest good, and the short-term desires possibly keeping you trapped and not moving forward to your goals as fast as you want. Perhaps it's the man or woman you know is not good for you but you spend time with them anyway because it's fun in the short term, but you are sabotaging your true desires of finding a romantic partner or good friends who are in alignment with your greater vision. Or you really want to buy the girl guide cookies because they have those chocolate mint ones you love and hey, it's supporting a good cause. But you are twenty pounds overweight and you know you will feel terrible after you eat them, and you can't have only one when the whole box is available. You give in, support the good cause but harm your wellbeing and delay the goal you desire for your health. Short-term desires can be strong and they are not all bad. I'm not saying don't have fun or indulge a little bit, it's all about enjoying the journey, but keep those experiences in check and stay connected to your greater vision for your life by listening to your deepest truest heart always.

Prayer is the perfect partner to intuition.

If you ever feel sidetracked by any of the above or any other life circumstance or way of being, prayer can bring you back to center, reconnecting you with truth. Prayer is a simple and efficient way to cut through chaos. It's an intentional way of guiding your energy back to the Divine that is always present.

Prayer is the perfect aid to clarity in life. You can simply ask for the chaos to be cleared and to gain clarity and super-naturally, you will find it. It's not always instant but it definitely can be. A simple one-sentence prayer or a few minutes of devoted sharing and asking can make waves of clarity and confidence in your life possible whenever you need it.

A simple prayer to find peace and center in chaos may sound like this:

"Dear Divine, please help me see the truth and find peace within."

You can pray for guidance in the situations above regarding short-term desires and outer influences by saying this:

"Dear Divine, please show me how to navigate these desires for human connection, or sweets".

Take a brief moment to receive and feel the clarity. Perhaps you are guided to have a conversation with the person in your life you know isn't for your highest good, or you give the girl guides money to support their cause but don't take the cookies, or take them and share them at a special function to celebrate your healthy choices in loving yourself.

Simply put, prayer is a reconnection to truth. It can be simple or complex. I'm a fan of simple.

Saying your prayer out loud is particularly effective, though not necessary. It is a way of vocalizing the desires of the heart and strengthening the inside/outside connection in your world.

Prayer and meditation strengthen your wholeness. Prayer is a good way to anchor intention, cleanse your energy, release fear, and ask for healing. It doesn't have to look a certain way as we are all brilliantly unique. I remember growing up, my family always prayed before the evening meal, and read the Bible after. As we grew and became busier with after-school activities this tradition faded but I can see now how centering these practices were for us as a family.

Prayer is the perfect partner to intuition.

I like to say "Be Religious about your spirituality". It's not either/or, religion or spirituality. The word religion comes from the Latin word meaning "to bind", which is to stay connected. I have a belief in Christ and was raised in the Christian religion but have also seen this belief system go horribly wrong to the point where I found myself brainwashed by someone who might be labeled as a religious psychopath. That experience was terrifying and when I got out I was at rock bottom. I had more debt than I could handle, I was unemployed, homeless, and afraid of the dark. Finding myself here, after what started as a miraculous series of events that led to my brainwashing and giving my power away, I dedicated my life to discovering the truth about life, religion, and spirituality. Now I don't claim to have all the answers but it fascinates me the way religion, spirituality, and science are now all coming together.

Through my journey, I have grown in my understanding of different religions and paths to personal awakening, and I see the heart as the center of us, through which the Divine works, whatever label you may place on yourself. What you believe has a tremendous influence on your life so be diligent about the thoughts you think and the beliefs you own as yours. When I say be religious about your spirituality what I mean is to take it seriously to the extent you are comfortable. It doesn't have to be your whole life, but it is a part of your life as a whole. There truly is no separation. You don't need a religion or to go to a specific building or place to worship the beauty of life and creation. If you do that is wonderful. Keep it rooted in love and peace, strive for personal growth, and the betterment of all.

Last but certainly not least in this chapter on faith and intuition is FUN! This is serious work but don't take it so seriously that you forget to have fun with it.

"*Lighten up Buttercup!*"

Admittedly, this is my weakness. I was a painfully shy child and I tend to take life too seriously but I am working on it! After my father died, I was reading the book of funeral plans he had made for himself after his terminal diagnoses. Within it was a family tree and under my name it said...

"My daughter Vicki, takes life too seriously".

As I read this I thought, "you got me!" It was true! It hit me hard, and while taking life seriously has gotten me far, I am reminded to lighten up.

This lesson from my father further cemented when I spoke at his funeral a few days later. I kept my words brief as it was a difficult task and quite the contrast to speaking to 650 women at an empowerment seminar less than two weeks before. I planned to end my words with

"My father taught me what true love is and not to take life too seriously".

Standing in an elegant historic church in front of the large funeral attendance I spoke my final words as "My father taught me what true love is and not to take life too **damn** seriously!".

I instantly thought "Oops I said damn in church!" as I heard my father laughing, reminding me of his exact lesson, don't take it too seriously (even in church!), I took his lesson to heart and forward into my life.

What's it all for if you're not having fun? Be diligent about your growth and development, but don't block your joy. Once you are comfortable in yourself and energy mastery you will find creativity and self-expression are fun! I used to be afraid to express myself for fear of being shut down as I had been in the past. Now, years later having learned everything I am giving you in this book it feels good to express myself and be all I came here to be! People still try to shut me down, but I am rooted in my center and connected to my joy. Train yourself with seriousness, and seriously trust yourself, AND enjoy the ride along the way!

Your foundation is complete! You've learned about energy and have gentle awareness that allows you to make deep lasting change. You are nourishing your body for radiance, you've mastered your self-talk, and are following the voice of your soul! In part two we will build on this foundation and embody all you are made to be in this life. You will learn how to own your boundaries, take care of your precious vehicle for this life, your body, and how to maintain your center and calm through any life storm.

Part Two: Embody All You Are Made To Be

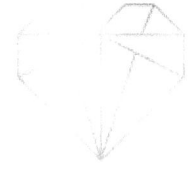

Chapter 5

Own Your Boundaries

Boundaries rock.
They help you claim your energetic sovereignty.

Boundary: something that points out or shows a limit or end; a dividing line (Merriam Webster)

"Personal boundaries are guidelines, rules, or limits that a person creates to identify reasonable, safe, and permissible ways for other people to behave towards them and how they will respond when someone passes those limits." -Wikipedia

It takes courage to first find and then enforce your boundaries. Boundaries start with ownership of your personal power which comes from within. Not in a bossy or uncaring way, but using your unique soul force from a place of grace so you have space and stamina to be your absolute best.

Without boundaries you will never get everything done that is important to you. Having rock-solid boundaries that flex when needed comes from a true connection to and knowledge of yourself. If you've lost that connection it can take some time to nurture it back into place and this book has lots of ways to help you get there. If you've already got that connection this chapter will back you up and support you in owning all of your power for the rest of your life.

Having boundaries is an act of self-respect. When you respect yourself, people automatically respect you more. Boundaries are what integrity is made of. It's not just about having boundaries with people outside of yourself, but it's also about the boundaries you cultivate within.

From an energetic perspective, boundaries provide the way for how energy flows into and through your life. Boundaries are like the bank of a river, allowing the life force energy (water), to flow towards freedom and ideal outcomes (the ocean).

When you know your boundaries and own them, you can be more productive, you know how you work best and what tasks to outsource. When you have clearly defined boundaries you can easily recognize when you are being drained energetically and find the source of the drain and fix the problem sooner rather than later.

I went through life not knowing my boundaries and wound up giving my power away over and over again. This left me feeling lifeless and wondering "what am I doing wrong?"

As I got to know myself and what I stood for I became more comfortable defining my boundaries and communicating them both verbally and non verbally. I became gracious about standing in my power and speaking my truth without the fear of being shut down or accused of being a bitch.

Having strong and clear boundaries is NOT about staying inside your comfort zone. It is about recognizing your limits and structuring your life in a way that allows you to stretch and grow while maintaining your high standards for yourself. Boundaries are about what you will and will not accept in your life. Yes, you will have to make compromises but you should know those things that you simply will not compromise on. For me, it's my health. I am in touch with my body to the point that when I get off track, my physical body will have none of it, and gives me a clear message to get back on track. If I ignore those messages, my inner voice and feelings get even stronger. My internal boundaries and standards for my health are so well established that my entire being will not settle for anything less than what supports these boundaries. This can make relationships tough at times when our society celebrates achievements, milestones, and even Friday nights with health-depleting foods. If you're having a birthday and someone offers to make you a cake it can be hard to decline if they are doing it out of love for you. But you must begin to speak up. I'm not saying never have cake; I love cake too. It's about habits and lifestyle. You wouldn't set a goal to lose twenty pounds and then start dating someone who is not on the same page, who drinks every night and eats junk food every day. Or maybe you would and you would overwrite those goals with poor habits. I've been guilty of this in the past, but eventually, it caught up with me. Lifestyles didn't match up and my body and soul wanted to get back on the path to health A.S.A.P.! Those relationships never last long because they are out of alignment for me.

Boundaries can be hard to maintain when you don't communicate WHY they are important to you and what all parties involved get out of it. For example, if you are trying to maintain a healthy lifestyle but a loved one continues to bring junk food into your home you may need to have a conversation that lets everyone know why it is important for you to be healthy and get them to support you. You would say first why it is important to you; you feel healthier, and you have more energy, which leads you to be kinder to your loved ones and not secretly upset with them for bringing the junk around. They in turn will also be happier and healthier in the long run. Therefore, it's win-win-win for you to be healthy. That is a practical example. Now let's get into the nitty-gritty energetic empowerment side of boundaries and how they are involved in energy mastery.

Let's start with your aura. Your aura is the energy field around your body. With my keenly trained intuitive senses, I can see others' auras, which appear different for everyone. They are different shapes, sizes, and colors. Your aura can get muddied up through the days or years if you don't master your energy. Mastering your energy will make your aura strong, a force of love to impact others.

Your aura is the energy of your being radiating out past your body. When you are in your authentic power your aura can be both a shield for you and a force of love you put out into the world. It can be a shield or act as antennae to help protect you. When you are fully in touch with yourself you can feel the world around you at deeper levels and you easily pick up on things that are in and out of alignment with your highest good. Have you ever had the experience of walking into a room and feeling good or bad energy? That's a combination of your intuition and your aura reacting to the environment. As you consciously strengthen your heart, your aura becomes stronger and you can then begin to shift the energy of places you go without having to think about it too much. Your energy leaves an imprint wherever you go so make it good.

On the flip side, you are also being impacted by energy everywhere you go. This is why energy mastery, knowledge of self, and strength of your heart are crucially important. Your aura can be impacted by things like blunt trauma, your level of enthusiasm or shyness, and many other factors. Your goal isn't to have the biggest aura or the strongest, but the one that is a reflection of your love. I know it may seem like I've gone off the deep end from the practicality of the book so far but stay with me. What is to come, even though it is more spiritual and energetic, will leave you pleasantly surprised and often wowed at how practical it becomes in your everyday life. This "woo-woo" stuff is key to your self-awareness and mastery so take a deep breath.

Inhale.........................exhale...............................

Open your mind and heart, and keep reading.

Now that you've opened your mind and heart to what's to come you are going to cover the basics of the chakras. Some people scoff when I talk about chakras, but lately I find most people are curious about what's happening in society and on the planet. Humanity is becoming more open-minded and looking for something greater. The chakra system is a great place to begin increasing your spiritual understanding which leads to greatness in energy mastery.

Diving into the chakras now let's discuss what they are and what they are not. Chakras are the main energy centers of your body. There are seven main chakras and many additional chakras throughout and around your physical body. Chakra means "wheel" and is a spinning wheel of energy that flows life force energy through you.

Chakras are not to be taken as some pseudo-religion or the be all end all of energy, but it is helpful to have a basic understanding and awareness of them. Knowing this information can change your life if you've struggled with a certain area of your body. The seven main chakras represent different stages of growth and different areas of life. When you become aware of these areas in your body you can notice more quickly when you are out of balance by how you feel within these centers.

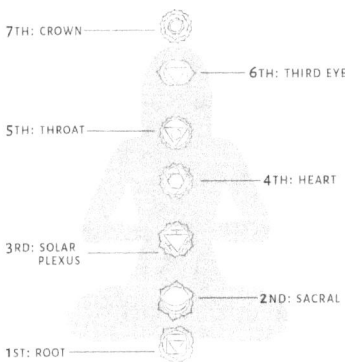

When discussing the chakras, refer to the base or bottom chakra as the first chakra, and the crown or top chakra as the seventh chakra. As you grow from infant to adult you are both living in and developing each energy center and this can have a big impact on how you go through life.

Beginning at infancy you are developing the first or root chakra which is all about safety and security. It is important to be held as a baby or this energy center may be off and you may have an imbalanced sense of safety and security in life. Moving up through the chakras you grow into your life with the development of the crown chakra which is about spiritual connection and trust in the Divine and your highest path. I will now discuss each of the chakras in more detail. See if you can understand how they relate to each stage of life.

Root Chakra

The root chakra is located at the base of your spine. The color normally associated with it is red.

This energy center is related to your sense of safety and security in the world. It is also your connection to the Earth. A balanced chakra will manifest in life as being grounded and having a solid foundation both within and outside of yourself.

When this chakra is off balance you may feel generally unsafe to explore the possibilities in your life or veer off the path of what you think others expect of you. You may put your trust in outside sources instead of placing trust in yourself and your abilities and resourcefulness.

Take a deep breath right now down into the base of your spine and visualize the color red. Take a few deep breaths and ask for nourishment and harmony to come to this part of your body. If you generally feel unsafe or are looking to make big leaps in your life, this is a good grounding practice to keep you rooted in your center as you take those steps. I like to think of it as my humanity, when I breathe into my lowest energy center it helps bring me back to earth, puts me fully in my body so I can take fully embodied actions towards my fulfillment.

Sacral Chakra

The sacral chakra is located below the navel in the body. The color normally associated with it is orange. This energy center is related to your creativity and self-expression in life. It is also linked to finances and communication which come from your creativity and expression. This chakra is also related to your divine feminine nature (which both men and women have) and is reflective of how you flow with life.

A balanced chakra will manifest as easeful digestion of both food and life circumstances, the ability to communicate and express yourself freely, and feeling in tune with the greater picture of your life and your purpose.

When this chakra is off balance you may feel disconnected from life, feel blocked from being able to create, or feel like you are stuck in relationships or jobs that don't serve your divine expression. You may feel bloating or stomach aches if you hold onto your words and ideas due to fear of being found out or put down for your ideas or for who you truly are (an ancient fear that is being cleared on the earth right now).

Take a deep breath right now deep into your belly. Visualize the breath turning orange and nourishing the area below your belly button. Ask for your creativity and expression to be harmonized in service and let go of any stagnant energy or fear. Take a few more breaths into this area and if you have space give your belly a gentle rub and thank it for all it does for you.

If you have struggled in this area, as I have, start a weekly or daily practice of rubbing oil on your belly and feeling grateful for it. This can help you start to get comfortable with all of you and support your divine self-expression.

Solar Plexus Chakra

The solar plexus chakra is located near the bottom of the rib cage in the center of your torso. The color normally associated with this chakra is yellow. This energy center is related to your power. It is related to the masculine aspect of yourself which is directly related to how you take action in life.

A balanced chakra will manifest in life as having strong personal boundaries and a clear mission you stand in and can speak about with ease. When this chakra is in balance you feel confident naturally and know you are in alignment and that your aligned actions serve the betterment of all.

When this chakra is off balance you may have low self-esteem and look for appreciation and acceptance outside of yourself instead of giving it and radiating it to and from your true self. As you align with your soul force you may notice some aches or discomfort in this area of your body as old patterns of twisting your power unravel.

Take a deep breath right now into your solar plexus which is the center of your body between the belly button and the lower ribcage. Visualize the color yellow and ask to be aligned with your divine love. Keep breathing deeply into this area and see yourself standing in your power, radiating your love and purpose into the world. Now ask for the right action steps to take or a simple insight into how you can use your power for good. Breathe deeply and gently as you receive your answer. If you don't hear anything it's ok! Breathe, visualize the color yellow, and ask for inner alignment, and to be made aware in the coming days and weeks of what personal power means to you.

This is also a great journal prompt; what does personal power mean to you?

Heart Chakra

The heart chakra is self-explanatory; it is located in the center of your chest and is the center of the seven main chakras. The color associated with the heart is green. This energy center is your connection to your soul, the source of your light which is the same source of all light and love. When you surrender to and open your heart, you live a life of passion and service, whilst at the same time feeling fulfilled and able to receive love from others and the Divine.

A balanced heart will manifest in life as being able to both give and receive equally in life. You know who you are as a child of God and you are worthy and deeply loved regardless of outer circumstance.

When your heart is off balance you may start conflicts in relationships as a result of being triggered. (This can happen even in the most loving relationships, relationships magnify your experience). You may cut yourself off from giving or receiving freely, feeling unworthy to receive which leads to a sense of lack. Or you hold back from giving your all for fear of being hurt, which is likely rooted in a childhood experience now locked in your nervous system or energy body.

Take a deep breath into your heart now and start by thanking your divine heart, simply for being. Breathe into your heart and visualize the color green. Feeling gratitude, invite your heart to gently open on the front, the back, the left, the right, top, and bottom. Opening your heart in all directions and feeling the energy of your heart begin to pour down your torso, legs, and arms. If it's comfortable to you, offer your day to your heart and ask it to lead the way forward. Breathe deeply. As you are feeling your heart make a commitment that you will remember to honour your heart each day.

When the heart is balanced and open, it is easy to maintain balance in all other chakras. Pay attention daily to your heart. Greet it each morning and ask it to guide your day. Thank it each night and pray for peace within. The heart is the center of your life, cultivate its glory.

Throat chakra

The throat chakra is located at the base of the neck. The color normally associated with this chakra is blue. This energy center is related to your communication and self-expression in life.

A balanced chakra will manifest in life as being able to speak your truth freely and easily. This goes for all areas of life from work, to family and friends, to your communication with yourself and your communication with the Divine. When your communication channel from the inside to the outside is free and clear you can stand up for yourself and others. It's not always easy. Sometimes you wait too long to say what you want or ask for what you need, but each of these awarenesses is an opportunity to practice using your inner voice to share with the outside.

When this chakra is off balance you hold back, swallow your words, and don't speak up when you know you should or even when you simply want to. You may get a frequent sore throat or have a sense of heaviness or tightness in the throat or jaw. Grinding your teeth can be a manifestation of holding back words, tears, or any emotions. As you release these old built-up energies you set your voice and the physical apparatus of the throat, neck, and jaw free.

Take a gentle long slow breath now and visualize the color blue, perhaps a sparkling royal blue ribbon wrapping itself and its healing energy around your throat and neck. See this gentle blue healing energy permeating your throat and neck gently re-aligning your throat chakra. See any old energies of pent-up emotions or words being released. You may need to sigh or vocalize, allow yourself the freedom to do it. If you need more time later to get to space where you can let out whatever is being released be sure to do that. Whether it is a scream or words that need to be said, know that releasing them in a sacred space where you are comfortable will not harm anyone but be released and transformed for the highest and best good of all. Breathe deeply and ask for your communication to be aligned with the message of your heart. Singing, chanting, humming, etc., regardless of if you think you can sing or not, has an exquisite healing effect on your throat chakra.

Sometimes when you begin using your voice to express your truth you may find you encounter resistance, inside and/or out. As I started aligning with my message, I began to plan my first live event. I felt wonderfully excited! I was going to teach a two-hour workshop on connecting with your inner wisdom. I worked diligently to create the content and prepare the materials. I set the date, booked the venue, and began promoting the event and selling tickets. Shortly into this process, under two weeks before the event, I came down with the nastiest cold I can ever remember having. It took me about eight days to recover. Only one piece was missing from my recovery, my voice!

I couldn't speak louder than a whisper right up until the morning of the event. In my heart, I knew not to cancel the event as I trusted my voice would return on time. Thankfully it did. My event went on wonderfully for the fair souls who showed up. I now recognize the voice loss as a manifestation of the fear I had around the importance of my voice and how strongly I felt called to use it to uplift and empower others.

As I have continued offering events and improving my self-expression I have had similar challenges but each time I followed through, the challenge became weaker and weaker. The next time I was to speak was at the Spring Festival of Awareness in the breathtaking Okanogan Valley of British Columbia. I had the chance to speak briefly to the entire conference delegation the opening evening, and then to a smaller group of about fifteen at my three-hour workshop entitled "Step Into Your Power".

The day before the event I began feeling a tickle in my throat. I spent the entire night diving into my internal energy and soothing my inner child, the part of me who was feeling fearful of being seen, sending her love in my heart and encouraging her greatness. Despite the lack of sleep, I got up ready to go with a full voice to share my message.

The point is, just because you hit some roadblock never means you should quit your dreams. You can take the lessons of the journey to fuel your growth and make you stronger. If I had canceled my events and not gotten out there and done my thing I would still have all of this in me to share, quite possibly driving me crazy.

When you encounter resistance, inquire and recognize it for what it is, and do the work to keep moving forward. This world needs you shining now.

Third Eye Chakra

The third eye chakra is located in the center of the head. The color normally associated with this energy center is indigo. This chakra is related to your ability to see things as they are and your connection and trust in your intuition.

A balanced chakra will manifest as having a clear vision for your life and being able to discern between what is good or not good for you. This discernment can be honed by asking yourself questions about the outcomes of different actions. For example, if I do this, what is a likely outcome, or what if I take this path instead? There is an interesting connection between the third eye and the solar plexus; your third eye helps you with vision and the solar plexus helps you take action and maintain boundaries to stay on your path to achieve your vision.

When the third eye chakra is off balance you feel like you are going through the motions of life. There may be a lack of passion if you feel like you "have to" do certain things to maintain your life instead of opening up to the possibilities and small action steps to create what your heart truly desires, the greater vision for your life. You may suffer from headaches or generalized confusion or possibly depression and anxiety.

Take a deep breath into your head and visualize the color indigo. Allow the breath to dissolve and remove any dissonant energy from this area, releasing it for cleansing. Breathe and allow yourself to witness yourself sitting by a river, allowing all of your thoughts to be absorbed and taken away by the water. Breathing and letting them go. Continue to breathe and ask to be shown a vision of your life where you are aligned, and allow the feeling of that to come into your mind's eye. It may even trickle into other areas of your being. Allow what will come to come, no forcing necessary. You may wish to journal about your experience after.

Crown Chakra

The crown chakra is located above your head. The color normally associated with it is violet. This energy center is related to your access and connection with higher consciousness and the Divine.

A balanced chakra will manifest in life as trust in oneself as well as the Divine in all areas of life. You understand there is a bigger picture and when you stay in a state of gratitude for this alignment and connection you manifest more goodness onto the earth. When the crown chakra is balanced you can access pure positive energy and invite it down through the crown into the rest of your body for healing and clarity.

When this chakra is off balance you feel cut off from anything sacred or divine. You may feel like life is only physical and there truly is no meaning to any of it (HINT: YOU get to CHOOSE the meaning of your life!) If the crown chakra is off balance you may feel tightness in the neck as the top of the head is not open to receive all that is flowing to and through you all of the time. This can be rooted in asking for something from God as a young child and that prayer not being answered. You may turn away from the Divine when you don't get what you think is best. As you grow and mature you can release your grievances with life and open to receive more insight and guidance.

Take a deep breath into your body and with the next breath bring your focus and the energy of the breath into the top of your head. Visualize the color violet. You may sense tingling or nothing at all. Ask to release barriers to Divine guidance. With the next few breaths let any old energy or ideas that no longer serve you go and notice how you feel throughout the rest of your day.

While the chakras are "separate" there is a lot of interconnection between them and how the energy flows in your being. When one is out of balance, the others can compensate, which throws them off balance as well. This is clear to see in people who don't feel secure in themselves (imbalanced/underactive root chakra), who feel the need to flaunt their power or use it to manipulate themselves, others, or who want to be significant (imbalanced/overactive solar plexus).

Another common connection is an imbalance between the throat and sacral chakras. If someone has trouble communicating and speaking their truth (imbalanced throat chakra), they are keeping their self-expression and creativity within which can lead to digestive upset (imbalanced sacral chakra).

I had this problem for much of my teenage years into my early thirties. I felt invisible and disconnected from my voice and often swallowed my words or kept my thoughts to myself. This manifested as chronic bloating and stomach pain. Over the years I learned to release the built-up energy in my sacral and solar plexus chakras and cleared the path between my heart and my throat chakras so I could communicate freely. What a profound difference this has made in my life! Before I easily shrunk back into my comfort zone and invisibility. Now I ache to speak and be seen for who I truly am so I can serve others at the highest level I am capable of. Occasions of bloating and stomach discomfort are rare now and when I do experience them I take it as a sign that I am not digesting something properly in my life or am holding myself back, which I can then take actions to remedy!

Take a moment to reflect on what you've read above. Take a few deep breaths and simply notice in your body any tightness or imbalances you can initially feel. There is no need to force healing or balancing of the chakras, simple love and breath can work miracles in your life.

Now that you are familiar with your chakras, let's return to your boundaries and see how it all comes together. The one area of your life that can have a mega impact on your energy is your boundaries. Not having strong boundaries can tear you apart energetically and spiritually. Without clear boundaries, you are constantly pulled in all ways by different people and situations in life.

Boundaries are limits that define acceptable behavior. Without boundaries, it is easy to become disconnected from your passion and purpose which come from within. Boundaries should make you strong, but also be flexible. Know yourself, know your limits, know what you are willing to do, and put up with, and what you are not. Without strong boundaries, you can waste years of your life giving in ways that drain you. With strong boundaries and a connection to your true self, you can be of service and give in ways that feel good and elevate you while serving and uplifting others.

How do you establish clear boundaries? You have to begin by knowing what you want and need. This comes from knowing yourself and having a clearly defined vision. Then you need to communicate these wants and needs both verbally and nonverbally. Your communication channel, the flow between your heart and your throat that comes out as words must be strong or exercised to become strong if at first it is weak (mine certainly was!) It can help to get a deep energy clearing and have someone such as myself guide you through a reconnection to yourself to begin establishing or maintaining boundaries that have been broken. Sometimes simple rest is the first step because we are overworked and stressed out as a society and we forget who we are and what we want and need as spiritual beings.

Once you have established your boundaries you need some tools to maintain and restore them when they are stepped over. Stepping over boundaries can happen with people or situations outside of ourselves, or they can even happen within ourselves. In any case, be aware and take a few minutes to reestablish trust within yourself. Boundaries are the foundation of trusting yourself. I go much deeper into this topic and cover multiple tools for creating and maintaining boundaries, as well as personal energy clearing and mastery techniques in my program Clear Confidence Energy Mastery.

The key way to maintain and restore boundaries is to have a clear vision and remind yourself of it often. There is a reason why you want to have your goals written down and in front of you as much as possible. When you know where you are going you tend to get there. If you don't have goals or know where you are going it is easy to squander precious time and energy and never get anywhere. My hunch is if you are still reading this book you have a vision deep within your heart wanting to manifest. Listen to it, create an external reference of it such as a vision board or goal statement, and remind yourself often of the truth that this is who you already are (more on this in the following chapters).

When you get off track or feel thrown off-center make sure you breathe deeply and visualize white light running down through your body and down into the earth, clearing and strengthening your entire energy field. This is an easy way to ground and center yourself and re-establish your boundaries.

Sometimes if you have had an intense energy exchange with another person (family, friend, colleague, customer or even a total stranger), you may have an entanglement with their energy. If you feel unclear simply ask the Divine to cut any energetic cords or attachments between you and that person or all people you interacted with that day. When you have entanglements with others it can be difficult to remain sovereign and true to ourselves. Please don't get this confused with cutting people out of your life or being cold and harsh to them. This is an energetic technique to keep you connected with the love that you are. Freeing yourself from other's energy makes you stronger and more capable of truly loving others and creating win-win relationships. At any time you can release other's burdens or energies into the earth or back to the Divine for healing, for the highest and best good of all.

If you find you get entangled with others' energy often, pay attention to that. Remember that awareness is the first and most important key to energy mastery. Perhaps you are an empath, or sensitive, and easily get roped into helping others, but don't empower yourself in the process. I used to do this all the time.

As an empath myself, people are drawn to me. Total strangers come up to me in public places and tell me their deepest darkest secrets and leave feeling refreshed and clear. It's a divine gift I have and I used to go along with it without thinking about how I could be of greater service. Eventually, I learned to master my energy so this experience didn't drain me. I knew there was more I can give than to absorb others' pain for them. I began to open my heart to the divine and transmute the energy I was absorbing into light by sending it into the earth and asking for it to be cleansed and cleared for the highest and best good of all.

This is a simple prayer you can use to clear your energy, maintain and restore your boundaries:

Dear Divine, Please cut any cords, remove any attachments, and clear my energy field of anything that is not love. Please send this energy into the center of the earth for cleansing, clearing, and transmutation for the highest and best good of all. (And visualize this happening as you say it.)
Thank you. Thank you. Thank you. (And breathe!)

I like to visualize pure white light for a moment after this prayer to bring me back to focus.

If the spiritual content of this chapter feels like too much, take what resonates with you and leave the rest. And if you're curious, give it a try. You've got nothing to lose except any low vibrational energy which doesn't serve you anyway.

Over time as you begin to own and understand your boundaries you will get stronger. During this process (and all of life is a process), you can start to track when and where you lose your power. With what people and in what situations do you feel drained or get off track with your goals and vision? As you recognize these patterns you can start to deconstruct them and build new ones into your life. The same goes for habits.

The first step is awareness, then you interrupt the pattern by calling it in and calling all of you in. (I say calling it "in" instead of calling it "out" because when it comes to transformation you must embrace your full experience with love and using the word "in" is inclusive, whereas "out" is exclusive. Give it a try next time you want to call someone "out", change your language to calling them (or you) "in", and feel the difference.)

Next, remind yourself of your goals and take one small action to work towards them and over time those unsupportive patterns lose their grip. You become stronger and more connected to your truth than ever before as you speak inwardly and out loud about what you want and need.

Boundaries are not about shutting others out of your life. Boundaries enhance relationships. Healthy relationships are interdependent, not codependent. Codependent relationships are where two people rely on each other for fulfillment instead of realizing fulfillment is an inside job. This creates a vicious cycle of trying to get happiness from another. It can feel nice in the short term but is disastrous for long-term relationships.

Interdependence is enhanced when each individual's independence is based on respect for self and others. Having strong boundaries is an act of self-respect. It allows you to honor and lift yourself up every day which gives you the strength to honor and lift others up. This is true for all kinds of relationships, from friendships, romantic relationships, family, and colleagues. When you have clear boundaries you show up and bring your best self forward.

Once you understand and are in tune with your boundaries, it's important to know and recognize how they are different from your comfort zone. Boundaries are a way to protect yourself and keep you safe, yes, but from a place of self-knowledge and self-respect. Boundaries are inner lines of what you will accept as your standards. Boundaries also propel your growth into your greatness as you continually come back to these standards and reach for your most fulfilled life every day. Boundaries help you stay on track. For example, if it's a health goal, the boundary is to respect the body and not indulge in more than two of grandma's amazing cookies. It's ok to eat the cookies but not so many you make yourself sick.

Comfort zones keep you where you are.

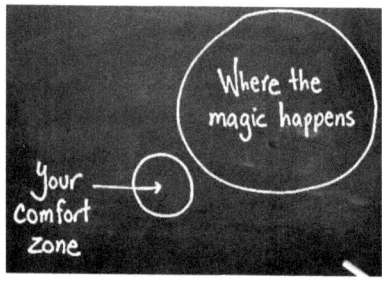

Comfort zones may feel nice but if you're reading this book I bet you are looking for more, and now you know that the growth zone is outside of your comfort zone. Boundaries help protect you when you are in the growth zone so you don't get taken advantage of by scam artists or burn yourself out by growing too fast.

You will notice when you step out of your comfort zone that a small part of you, the survival mechanism of your brain will try to sabotage you, take you out and tell you all sorts of nasty things to bring you back into the comfort zone. Be aware of this reaction, it can be loud or quiet. Mine tends to be quite loud. When I stepped into a bigger game and started making and sharing videos and content from my place of purpose, my survival brain always stepped in after I put something out into the world. My survival brain is full of fear of what other people will think, and JUDGEMENT! It told me all sorts of things about how I look and the information I put out. It was so nasty it made me want to hide in a cave for the next two years! But I didn't let it. In those circumstances, I recognized the voice of the survival, or lizard brain (mentioned in chapter four). I reminded myself of who I truly am (Grace, Love, Power, Resilience, Home) and claimed that. I encouraged my inner child to be free and reminded myself that I am safe. I'm not going to die from putting a video out! Over time, the voice of fear and judgment got quieter as I built new habits and expanded my comfort zone to include being visible.

The survival brain is tricky and it's not going anywhere soon. You must learn to recognize its voice and stand strong in your truth and authenticity when it shows up. When you step outside of your comfort zone it will show up. It is pretty much guaranteed. But you don't have to succumb to its voice. Breathe deeply into your heart, remind yourself of who you are, voice your goals out loud, and take one small action step toward them.

As you grow, your awareness and connection to your true self is the basis of your energy mastery. Personal energy and boundary awareness are parts of life you can integrate firmly in your being so you don't need to study this stuff forever. It is important to review and have some coaching and healing guidance along the path, but once you have these main understandings and integrations you will be a hundred times farther ahead than those who don't. When you have this information and integration you can follow your heart to embody all that you came here to be.

In the next chapter, you will learn how important taking care of your physical body is to personal power and energy mastery.

Chapter 6

Love Your Body

Looking good and feeling good go together. You cannot separate the mind, body, heart, and spirit, although many people try to. Or, as in my case, forget about one of these aspects. Growing up as a girl, I focused way too much on my physical body. I didn't realize how much my mind was controlling me and saying terrible things about myself, and I completely shut down my spiritual life in an attempt to hang out with the cool kids who all became atheists. As you can imagine, not being true to myself led to all sorts of problems, which eventually led to my journey of integrating all aspects of me back into wholeness. I now teach these wholeness principles as a part of the foundation of energy mastery.

Right after my university degree in Health Promotion, I became a Certified Personal Trainer and attempted to make that my career. What I found was this was only one step in my journey to energy mastery. As I grew, I uncovered that we cannot only focus on our physical bodies when we think of health. This chapter focuses on the physical aspects of exercise and we'll weave in how this affects your mind and spirit.

Looking good and feeling good go together, and the easiest way to realize this is with regular exercise. Your body is what you get to take action with. Exercise, as much as it burns energy and calories, also produces more long-term sustained energy for you.

When you feel good and look good you can begin to use your ego to drive your health results. The ego loves to look good and feel good and if you can see this from a higher perspective you can use your ego, instead of having your ego use you. Let the ego's insatiable desire for significance drive the sustained health practices in your life. Not to the detriment of over-exercising, restricting calories, or putting yourself down, but allowing the ego to cause you to make better choices. Overall, your choices must come from your heart but you can get your ego in service to the bigger health picture.

Energy mastery requires exercise as a regular habit. Not something that gets done once in a while, but a fully ingrained habit that is a part of who you are. So much so, that when you don't exercise you feel drained, or your body begins to crave movement. The bare minimum you should work out is three times a week. If you currently do no exercise, start with one or two times a week and work your way up from there. If you are already at four to seven days a week you are phenomenal, keep up the good work! How can you switch it up or challenge yourself this week?

If you're newly getting into working out it's helpful to have rituals or triggers for exercise. For example, maybe you exercise first thing in the morning, or right after work each day. These triggers or set times condition your mind and body to desire exercise at those times. My chosen time to work out is in the morning before I do anything else. But somedays it doesn't work and I end up working out in the evening. This is ok as long as I am doing it! Start where you are and grow from there.

Exercise means cardio, strength, and flexibility training.

Cardio exercise is what gets your heart and blood pumping! Think of running, swimming, sports like soccer or basketball or anything that makes you go fast. The effort put into cardio exercise creates blood flow in the body, it causes your breathing rate to increase which oxygenates your blood and body and leads to more energy over time. (Even if you are wiped out after your workout!). Cardio is great for burning calories, reducing stress, and strengthening the cardiovascular system. (more heart love ♥)

Strength training is using either body weight or other heavy things to strengthen your muscle tissue. All people need strength training. Men are generally comfortable lifting weights but women tend to shy away from this part of the gym which is a huge mistake! Women often believe they will get big and bulky when they lift weights when the truth is, for most women, lifting weights only sculpts and tones your body, helping you stay lean.

Strength training, or resistance training, is one of the few areas in life when resistance creates growth. When you lift weights or do other forms of strength training you are using the resistance to create growth in the muscle tissue. This is good because muscle burns more calories than fat! Don't be afraid to work on those muscles! This is especially important as you age. Strength training helps maintain your strength and independence. Strength training keeps the body strong and helps you age well. Strength training is not just for your muscles, it also protects your bones and can slow or prevent the onset of osteoporosis.

Last, but certainly not least, is flexibility. Now here we are talking about physical flexibility, but this ties into your ability to be flexible in all areas of life, which is why it is so important. Flexibility is gained by stretching your muscles. Stretching promotes relaxation and helps your muscles recover after intense or even gentle workouts. When you are flexible you are less prone to injuries and you reduce post-workout pain. Always stretch after you exercise and perhaps enjoy a nice relaxing stretch before going to bed at night to help you relax.

Combining all three, cardio, strength, and flexibility gives you the foundations of exercise. You can incorporate all three separately into your life such as running, weight lifting, and stretching. Or you can find certain activities that combine all three such as yoga, or a Barre style class.

Cardio helps keep your heart strong. The focus that exercise requires keeps your mind sharp. Flexibility helps reduce and prevent pain and strain. Exercise helps you maintain your health as long as possible.

Whatever your current physique, and whatever you want to achieve, when you take care of yourself you look and feel your best. When you exercise your clothes fit better, you have healthier percentages of fat and muscle, and you gain natural confidence through movement. If you're feeling stuck in a rut, try out a new routine, or join a new class to shake things up. There are countless ways to grow as a person inside and out but the last thing you want to do is not have time for your health. If this is an issue let's connect and find something that works for you. Your health is far too valuable to get swept under the rug.

> ***"The greatest wealth is health."***
> Virgil

Your exercise routine must be enjoyable for you. If you hate going to the gym, chances are that buying a membership and forcing yourself to go will be one of the most difficult things you do. It doesn't have to be this way! You may need to try a few things before you find the exercise groove that suits you. It has to be fun. You want to be exercising because you love yourself and it feels good, not because you ate too much, or as a form of punishment. If you find something you love you will find you keep going back for more. Some people love the dancey grooves of step class or Zumba. Me, I'm not co-ordinated like that. Those classes look fun but are like torture to me! I prefer to shake my booty and let loose in the living room. If you find something you love you can connect with others who also love that thing which builds community. All of these things are great for mental health too! Taking care of your body isn't just for the body, it is for all of you, and you are magnificent.

Sometimes you can't do it on your own, you need support. This is when the buddy system comes in. Having someone on your side encouraging you, and keeping you accountable enhances your chances of success in any area of life. Some days you may not feel like going for a walk, but your buddy can hold you to it and vice-versa.

Your workout buddy can push you in ways maybe you couldn't, and when it comes to exercise, pushing yourself is very important! Remember when you were pushed as a child, gently, or not, by a teacher or parent/guardian to do something new? They pushed you past your comfort zone so you could grow as a human. I remember hating this, throwing tantrums, and being terrified to do something new that seemed unusual or unnatural to me. Most of the time though, on the other side of doing the new thing, I felt amazing, like a superhero who could do anything! It's the same as an adult. Often when we are done school we lose touch with the growth cycle and can find ourselves settling into a mediocre life. There's nothing wrong with this per se but my guess is if you are reading this book you are looking for more. More comes from pushing yourself past your comfort zone, in exercise, and all areas of life. The goal is to never stop growing.

As you push yourself, you become stronger and faster by breaking through preconceived limits and barriers, and therefore your previous benchmarks. Think you can only run five miles? Push yourself to run seven, and then ten. Think you can only lift twenty-five pounds? Push yourself to lift thirty, and then thirty-five. You get the point. Go a little bit "Harder, Faster, Stronger, Longer" and see how you feel both physically and mentally.

If this is hard to do on your own, and the buddy system doesn't work for you, hire a trainer! Effective trainers (and coaches) will lovingly kick your ass and you will be better for it. This isn't your school bully, but someone who is pushing you and supporting you in your goals. Trainers are professionals who help you break through your limits in the name of greater health and wellness. They will push you past what you think you are capable of and that alone is worth the investment. Even if you think you can't afford a trainer but feel it would be of benefit to you, do some research. See what the actual cost is. Interview some trainers to see how they would help you. You will gain some insight and motivation from talking to them, and you may find you have the willingness to invest once you get a sense of the possibilities. Some trainers have group or family options to help you lower the price. The point is, get your ass kicked and see how good you feel after.

If this chapter is rubbing you the wrong way, see how you can step back and reframe your relationship to exercise. How can it feel good for you? If what I'm saying anywhere in this book doesn't resonate with you, ask yourself why then ask yourself what will work for you? Your inner voice is most important but knowledge and science have pieces of the puzzle.

I mention breathing and its importance a lot in this book. Exercise pretty much forces you to breathe which is fantastic for energy mastery. As your lungs are working, all the old air is being forced out and new fresh air is being brought into your body. Sometimes you breathe shallow and don't get fresh air into the bottom of your lungs, exercise helps this. As you breathe deeply and oxygenate your blood, this also strengthens your heart which sends the blood around the circulatory system and oxygenates all of your tissues. This oxygenation leads to longer-lasting energy. Perhaps you've heard of "runners high" which is a sense of wellbeing that comes after exercise? This is due to endorphins; chemical hormones released by the endocrine system that help you feel good! It's a positive cycle; exercise makes you feel good!

Hopefully, by now you get that exercise is a key component of energy mastery but I wanted to bring it back to a statement I highly align with:

Exercise is only 20%, diet is 80%.

Going back to chapter two, you must fuel your workouts properly. Clean fuel and plenty of water help your systems run smoothly. If you exercise on junk food your recovery time will be slowed, and you won't have as much energy and clarity to make it through your workout.

Clean fuel = more energy for working out.

You must train your body to crave movement. This starts from the inside with seeing yourself as healthy, vibrant, and truly alive. When you can connect with this vision at the core of you (without faking or forcing, but knowing it as truth), then all of your thoughts and actions begin to come from there. When they don't, you catch them and reroute them back to the truth. Begin to cultivate your vision of yourself as healthy by seeing yourself as strong (in all areas of life), having fun, and feeling energetic. Begin within, begin where you are, begin now. You got this.

In the next chapter, you will learn how to fully root into your center and live from there through the incredible practices of breathing and meditation.

Chapter 7

Breathe and Meditate

Our attention span sucks.

With bright, flashy TVs, loud violent video games, constant reliance on technology, the attention span we have has shrunk and shrunk some more. I'm not knocking technology, it's been a great stride in evolution in many ways. However, when it is abused and used in ways that harm consciousness there needs to be another way.

Think about your own life; how long can you simply sit and be with yourself? No distractions.

Perhaps you have shiny object syndrome, going from one thing to the next, often based on simple short term desires, or thinking the next thing is what will finally do it for you, but then it doesn't, or you get bored quickly so you move onto the next thing. It's like a dog happily walking with its owner who sees a squirrel and runs away to chase it, leaving the owner in the dust. Your attention can get grabbed quickly by outside things when you are not focused. Your heart is always content to simply be, while your mind, left untrained, is running after what it believes is the next best thing. Buddhists have dubbed the mind that is unsettled, restless, and uncontrollable the "monkey mind".

If your "monkey mind" is out of control you must work on it, or it can destroy your dreams!

Your monkey mind is always going after what's next. Left untrained and unskilled in meditation, the mind is unfocused on where it is going. It has a total lack of discipline. This makes it so you rarely keep the promises you make to yourself.

For example, tomorrow I will go to the gym, or start my blog, or clean the excess out of my home.

Whatever you truly desire that will move you forward in life, your monkey mind is slippery and skilled at finding ways out of those things. The monkey mind goes after temporary pleasure only, which over time keeps you stuck where you are. This kills long-term true satisfaction in life.

Take a deep breath.

There is a chance your monkey mind is feeling distracted at this moment. If it is, take another deep breath and continue reading for more on how to master your energy and focus to create your dreams.

Meditation and breath are vital keys to energy mastery. They don't have to be difficult, but they can be challenging. Many people truly believe they cannot meditate. The truth is, anyone can do it, but it takes consistency and dedication. From an evolutionary standpoint, your senses are trained in protecting you. Loud noises and other senses distract you from your center and keep your attention on the outside world in a protective way. Combine this with modern technology that is shortening your attention span and lack of mental focus training and it's no wonder people find meditation hard. But let me tell you it is worth it! Even if meditation for you doesn't involve sitting still and watching your breath. Perhaps for you, it is focusing on one task at a time so you can finally complete it. If you get into a state of flow while working on your projects, that is a form of meditation. You can even be doing your job while meditating, but this often takes some training in silent meditation first.

When I first went on my search for spiritual truth, I meditated every day, morning, and night for at least twenty minutes for about two years. I have continually meditated since then but not always on the same schedule, and not always with the same technique. I've been to Vipassana retreats where you meditate for twelve hours a day for ten days straight, and many other meditation events.

If you think meditation is hard, ask yourself why you want to start meditating. Are you finding yourself worrying too much, or getting scatter-brained, or perhaps you want to listen to your inner voice more instead of the voices outside of you. Write your reason down and have it wherever you will do your meditation; on a cushion on the floor, next to the armchair, wherever. It could even be in your parked car. Decide which type of meditation you would like to do. Would you like to begin with a prayer to center yourself, or are you going to use a guided meditation? You get to choose. Start where you are and begin, this is the only way to overcome not doing it.

Meditation helps you reclaim your focus for the things that are truly important to you. Meditation is about connecting to you, so you don't get sidetracked constantly and end up wondering where your life went. I am a huge fan of simple breath-focused meditation since it is both the simplest and potentially the hardest but comes with phenomenal results.

My recommendation is based on what was recommended by an incredible healer who helped me jumpstart my spiritual journey after a traumatic experience. After our first eye-opening session, the healer asked me to begin a daily meditation practice which I will share with you. It had such a huge impact on my progress toward understanding myself, healing the trauma, and stepping into my power. The practice is simple, but don't let it fool you. It is serious mental training to get your monkey mind under control. It will help strengthen your mental focus and connection to your beautiful heart.

The goal is to do this meditation for twenty minutes twice a day. If that is too much, start lower with two to five minutes. If you can start at twenty that is best. Set your timer and don't move or open your eyes until it goes off. For that time sit comfortably and with your inner eye watch your breath moving in and out of your nose. Pay attention to the sensation of the breath moving in your nostrils and down your throat. Keep your attention here the entire time! Notice when your attention drifts, it certainly will. When you notice you are thinking about other things, gently bring your attention back to your breath. Do not entertain thoughts of what you can't do or how you got distracted or what the thoughts are about. This is only for twenty minutes! Bring your attention back to the breath, again, and again, until the time is up.

In the beginning, your mind will drift A LOT! This is normal. As you gently train your focus back to the breath it will become more natural. If it helps, you can bring one word into your mind to repeat. I'm a fan of the word "love" and thinking about the vibration or feeling of love while I repeat it in my mind.

Keep your focus on your breath, bring the attention back to the breath, and/or your word of choice. Over time you will be amazed at how much you can uncover energetically as you simply focus. The first ten minutes may feel like torture but keep at it and when the timer goes off you may be disappointed as you were melting into such bliss for the last five minutes. You will begin to notice your world becoming more colorful, and your intuition is heightened along with your new clarity and focus.

If the breath focus meditation seems like too much you can use technology to help (imagine that)! There are many apps and videos and music to help with meditation.

When I began this breath focus meditation practice I remember feeling my vibration raising the more I meditated. I was no longer distracted by my destructive thoughts, I was more in tune with myself, and this practice is what began to release my spiritual gifts, which by the way, everyone has.

Beginning a daily practice will train your focus. In the beginning, daily practice is a must for energy mastery. Daily maintenance will enhance your awareness in all areas of life and help keep you centered during times that may be unsettling. If it seems hard trust that it gets better with practice. Don't beat yourself up if you struggle- it's called "practice" for a reason!

Begin where you are and do what you can. The goal is twenty minutes twice a day. Watch your energetic awareness and mastery skyrocket with this practice! Over time you will find you can maintain your focus in your everyday life as your inner world of alignment begins to reflect in the outer world. You may drift from the practice over time, and that's ok. You may find new practices that suit you. That's ok. This practice is always impactful and something you can come back to. If you get to twenty minutes twice a day and over time you get busy and can only meditate once a week, so be it. You won't forget the connection you developed during your time meditating. Keep a consistency that works for you and maintain a practice of some sort over the long haul. Practices and habits come and go but once you've got this one ingrained it is like riding a bike; you never forget.

With daily practice and long-term implementation of meditation and breath focus, your connection to your true self will be so enhanced you may feel like a whole new person! When you quiet the mind, the heart speaks louder and more freely. Or maybe at the same pace and volume it always did, but now you can actually hear it! Daily quiet time will allow more truth to arise from within, pushing its way to the surface and clearing out old energy that may be keeping you stuck. With this deeper connection to yourself you have space for a deeper inquiry into life's most important and engaging questions such as "who am I?" and "why am I here?". The space you create through breath and meditation also allows more room for contemplation of the answers you receive and how to best act upon them. This all leads to you being all you are and all you came here to be!

~Start where the breath meets the heart.~

As an empath and healer, the call upon my heart and life is to lift others through the transmutation of energies. I use heart breathing to stay present and grounded in my daily life, as well as when I am guiding another. Heart breathing is something I picked up from my friends and mentors Patricia and Bill Clum at Evolution of the Heart.

Before meeting these wonderful souls, I did a lot of work; spiritual development, psychological and mindset work, health, and nutrition work. All this life-changing work was incredible, and I was diligent with it. What seemed to be missing was the deep soul integration of all the spiritual truths I learned about. It wasn't until I met Patricia and Bill that things truly started to change for me.

The many hours I have sat with Patricia and Bill consist of a lot of deep breathing, specifically to open the heart. The heart chakra is the center of your being. As a baby, you came into life open and bright but the world usually offers experiences of pain that may cause you to put up walls and barriers in trying to protect your sacred heart while you forget that you are love.

Through breathing deeply into the heart, you must face these walls and have the courage to open your heart once again. This often leads to emotional releases as stored energy and emotion finally have space to "breathe". Over time and practice with devotion to your soul, which you reach through the heart, you become stronger in your wisdom and knowledge of your true self.

Your heart is always calling and guiding your forward. Will you say "yes" and follow the call? Will you open your heart and mind, even deeper, and let in the grace of love? If you said "Yes!" your life may change in unforeseen ways. You may remember things you've previously forgotten, begin to release long-held emotions, and burst with beauty and joy because it is too much to contain. Let out all that your voice longs to express. No more holding back your voice- the voice of truth and love. I said "Yes" and the journey that has unfolded is more enthralling than I imagined. Having your body fully alive with the breath, self-awareness in tune, and a willingness to trust in yourself will take you farther than you ever dreamed.

Have you ever noticed when you are going through a stressful time that you hold your breath? This is a natural human experience but one that can cause problems over the long term. When you hold your breath you keep your energy stagnant. Did you know in the Hebrew language the word Spirit translates to breath? Breath is what you can use to bring energy to your body, mind, and spirit and when you hold it you are withholding nourishment from yourself.

On top of that if you hold your breath for too long while something stressful happens you can create energy blocks. These are places in your being where energy gets bound or stuck and may not move for a long time. Have you noticed in the wild when animals get caught off guard, fall, or go through a stressful event they shake themselves vigorously? This motion resets its nervous system and energy. What do we humans do a lot of the time? We go through something stressful and then we just keep going claiming to be "ok" or "fine" without moving the energy we've been holding or sit on the couch sulking waiting for it to pass. Well, you are an animal too and if you ever find yourself stressed out, simply notice, take a big breath, and shake it off. Notice how you feel after doing this.

At a dark time in my life, I met a charming and boisterous older gentleman named Frank who felt my sadness the first time I met him. We instantly became great friends and he was a trusted advisor to me for a short time before he passed on. He would often have me go out and hug a tree (nature is an amazing healer!) and shake my body out to get my energy grounded and moving. At his celebration of life, I met many other people who also met him in a dark time and he helped them in ways involving activities that seemed a little crazy to us in the beginning.

"In hindsight," one commented, "the shenanigans were a powerful way of shaking people up to wake them up and light the way out of the darkness."

I knew Frank was a special man right from the get-go but to hear all these similar stories cemented his Earth Angel status in my memory banks.

Resetting the nervous system with breathwork and movement is an amazing way to become centered, grounded, and beat energy blocks before they have time to set in. I will share many tools to get to the roots of blocks and how to clear them in future pages. Keep reading!

When it comes to deep breathing, I mean *really* deep breathing. Not just into your lungs, but all the way into your body. Basic breathing is not enough to relax the body and nervous system and affect yourself on an energetic level. You must take long slow deep inhales and exhales. Breathe in as much as you can, into your lungs, past your diaphragm, into your belly. See your breath filling your entire body even down your legs and arms. Obviously, you can't really get air into those areas but you can oxygenate the entire body via the blood and the power of visualization can enhance the deep breathing process. You must include your whole body as it is part of your entire being.

Invite and guide your breath into all parts of you. Into your fingers, toes, up into your brain and mind. If there is any tightness in your body, breathe into it. Simply breathing into it can begin to loosen the tight energy that is being held there. Breathing wakes up and brings consciousness into your body which enhances your experience of wholeness as a divine being. Without breath you die, so breathe! Become aware of the natural process of breathing, and bring deep conscious breathing into your life daily, especially when you are under stress. Deep breathing keeps you calm and connected.

Breathing is also an incredible process or tool to clear your chakras when you are having a particular challenge. Think back to the introduction to the chakras in chapter five. Consider if you are having a challenge in any particular area that could be associated with a chakra. You can breathe deeply into your chakra and visualize its color to help clear it out. You can also say some words of prayer or gratitude to help clear the chakra.

Breathe into one or all of your chakras. Invite them to open and release. You can even ask them for guidance, the same way you can for any area of the body that is feeling off. You know the phrase "ask and you shall receive"? It's also true for gaining answers from your physical being, and breath is the perfect partner to receiving your answers. I am a big supporter of doing a full chakra clearing because often when one is off balance another will compensate for it.

As wonderful as breath and meditation is for you in the now, it also has a massive impact on the bigger picture. The long-term impact of daily meditation practice and regular deep breathing is greater empathy with others. Through breathwork and meditation, you will have sourced the inner fountain of eternal peace you can connect with at any time. There will be less reliance on outside sources of temporary pleasure or surface-level fixes such as distractions or unnecessary medications with more negative side effects than beneficial health effects. You will have the ability to connect and stay true to your long-term vision which enhances mental health, personal relationships, boundaries, and the overall confidence to go for what you truly desire. You will have more clarity and be able to see the bigger picture in your own life, possibly as well as the bigger picture for others.

There are many different methods of meditation, and most of them are both relaxing and energizing. When you focus enough to relax into meditation, you drop all of the outside stressors weighing on you, which leaves you with more energy. Relaxing and energizing! Many techniques will help relax your nervous system and help you connect with the infinite source of energy within. Some of my favorite techniques other than simple breath-focused meditation are the breath of fire and progressive muscle relaxation. A simple web search will provide more detail if you are curious about those.

~Remember the sacred in each moment and breathe.~

Meditation and breathing are vital components to a life of short and long-term energy mastery. When you include these practices you get increased clarity and confidence. You will have more energy for your daily routine tasks, as well as the tasks that will take you out of your comfort zone and into the land of dream creation, not just dreaming. You will find old issues resolving themselves or showing you how to resolve them with grace. You will gain a greater understanding of yourself and others.

If you do nothing else from this book but a simple breath-focused meditation and take five long deep breaths every day you will be better off for it.

In this section, you learned how to own your boundaries, take care of your physical body for increased energy, and the critical importance of breathing and meditation. Now that you have your foundation and are embodying your power it's time for ongoing maintenance. Energy mastery is a lifetime experience that gets easier with practice. In section three you will learn how to truly forgive and let go so you can keep your energy clear from old energies that no longer serve you. You will discover how to overcome obstacles so you can achieve your heart's desires, the essential importance of your attitude, and how to never give up on what is truly important to you.

Part Three: Ongoing Maintenance

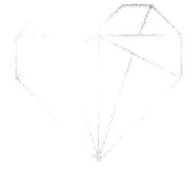

Chapter 8

Forgive and Let Go

*"Live and love fully with an open heart for all.
Give your love abundantly and enthusiastically.
Don't hold back.
Life is short, enjoy the ride."*

Frank

We all have bad things happen in our lives. What separates those who rise and those who stay stuck in the muck of the past is that those who rise know how to turn past experiences into fuel for the future. When you can forgive and let go, you engage your full potential.

My gift is helping people let go of what holds them back from expressing themselves more fully and to feel grounded and confident in their new expression. This is fascinating work because as human beings we are always evolving. Your life impacts you deeply and there is a lot of pain in the world, yet you don't need to hold onto the pain, stored emotions, and other blocks. This is truly an auspicious time where you can release these things and open once again to the love you are and must offer.

> "If you bring forth what is within you, what you bring forth will save you. If you do not bring forth what is within you, what you do not bring forth will destroy you."
>
> Gospel of Thomas

After studying, practicing, integrating, and teaching energy mastery for many years, I feel confident saying your open mind and willingness to discover new ways of being is the first step to mastering your energy. Curiosity creates openness in your being, which leads to expansion, fulfillment, and growth.

Even in times of sadness, stay present by using your breath. Be aware of how your emotions feel in your body. Asking for guidance, whether from the Divine or trusted others will make your journey much more meaningful. It will deepen your relationship with yourself, the Divine, and others in your life. And the deeper you are connected in these ways, the more ripples of presence, connection, and love flow out into the world, raising us all up.

Curiosity can open lines of communication in strained relationships and even help you make new friends. Curiosity is a great aid in the healing process. Instead of thinking you know something, allow the space for what's next to arise in truth, and shift you, as your awareness evolves.

Over the years I have thought I had all the answers or known the final truth. Through curiosity and dedication to truth, I have learned there are different truths in different times and for different people and that the only everlasting Truth is Pure Divine Love. Knowing this, it is my work to remove all barriers to Divine Love in my own experience. Uncovering, from the inside out, the Truth of who I am as a single expression of Divine Love. I remain unattached to any outcome but perhaps it will have a positive impact, somehow sometime. One of my favorite prayers that always ignites and opens my heart is "Dear Heart, show me the Truth."

Through my training and studying holistic health, science, energy medicine, and more I have learned so much! Through all of that, what I have witnessed as truth is;

Love heals. A message from my mentor's mentor I would like to share with you is "If all else fails, love them". I will add, if all else fails, love yourself. Truly, fully, unconditionally. Love yourself and your experience. Let love be the energy behind all you give. When you give from divine love you know it is a well that can never run dry. Give love liberally, to yourself first, then outward. Uncover all that prevents the free flow of love through your life and include it in the love. Melt distortions and shine a light on your fears. Invite more love in and through your life, always.

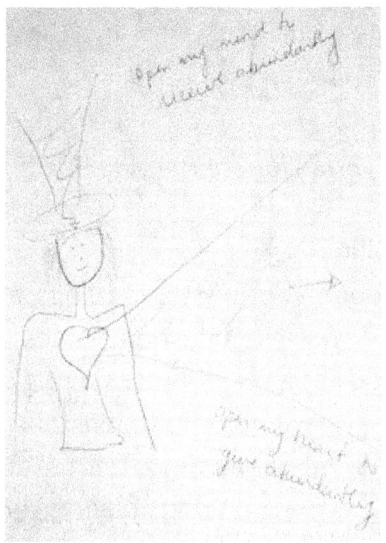

When I work with others, the main thing I see holding them back from experiencing this unconditional love and personal mastery is attachments to past ideas, experiences, and conditioning. I see this on the energetic level and work in that realm to help clear out this old energy and then coach my clients to become empowered in the now and to courageously create their future.

Transformation occurs when you morph the energy of pain into passion and then allow passion to drive you forward. It takes work, reflection, and insight.

A reminder:
Repression + Suppression = Depression

You must feel all of your feelings. Why is this so? Emotions are energy in motion.

Emotion = Energy in Motion

When you allow yourself to feel your emotions fully, they move through you. When you do not allow yourself to feel them, they stay stuck, sometimes settling within your energy body for years! Fully feeling your emotions is a major component of energy mastery. It's not about control, but about awareness, surrendering to your higher path, taking action, and having the tools to stay on the path regardless of outer circumstance or inner resistance. You are whole and feeling the full range of emotions is a part of wholeness. You must express yourself!

Emotional expression is the real spice of life.

Emotional blockages can get stuck in different areas of your body weighing you down over time.

When you permit yourself to feel all you are feeling and move the emotion through you, you set yourself free from any cages you have locked around yourself. Emotional expression is like releasing buried treasure from your emotional and energetic body. I now notice that when I do hold back from expressing myself I experience physical symptoms of discomfort and mental symptoms such as self-criticism. One time I held back from speaking my truth in a relationship and developed a rash on my throat! As soon as I shared my truth and ended the relationship it swiftly healed itself.

Many times, I have been blessed to sit in sacred space as I got in touch with my emotions that I used to label "bad" or "unacceptable" and began releasing them. Somewhere along my lifeline, I picked up the idea that I wasn't supposed to show my most intense emotions of anger, rage, sadness, grief, or even ecstatic joy. I made my emotions, and therefore myself, wrong. I put myself in a box and always tried to present myself as agreeable and "nice".

As I began noticing this, along with learning the value of releasing emotions, I had to practice the vulnerability of being seen in the process of emotional release. It wasn't easy, and it didn't happen all at once. I began noticing my "blood is boiling" when an emotion of anger wanted to express and release. I wrote pages and pages of angry notes to God, I screamed into a pillow with my door closed when no one was home. These practices began carving a pathway for the depth of my suppressed anger to finally be freed from within me and to feel safe expressing anger, and all emotions, as a part of a normal healthy human experience.

Eventually, being more connected with my truth from all the work before, I knew that anger wasn't me or who I am, and it didn't mean anything about me that I had these emotions. In the end, the clarity of wisdom that came from my soul, which was buried underneath the anger emotion was gorgeous. I was meant to experience anger as a fire fueling truth and action in my life! Suppressing anger doesn't help or protect others and left inside it only burns me.

When you have long-held emotions buried in your energy field they can create distortions that distract you from the truth of your wholeness. A piece of your consciousness is connected to the buried emotional energy and it can drain you of vitality. You've heard of "energy vampires", those people who seem to suck the energy right out of you when you hang out with them. Your buried emotions are like your own internal energy leech, but instead of being malicious, it is calling for loving attention. (Energy vampires themselves need love and attention, but like us, they need to give it to themselves first. They simply seek outside sources of love more fiercely than most).

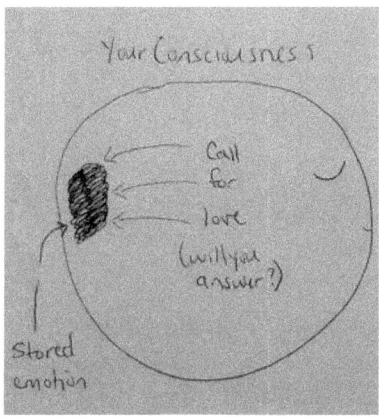

Sometimes, if you bury emotions too long the energy becomes dense. I don't know about you, but I like feeling clarity and confidence every day, I don't need heavy energies weighing me down.

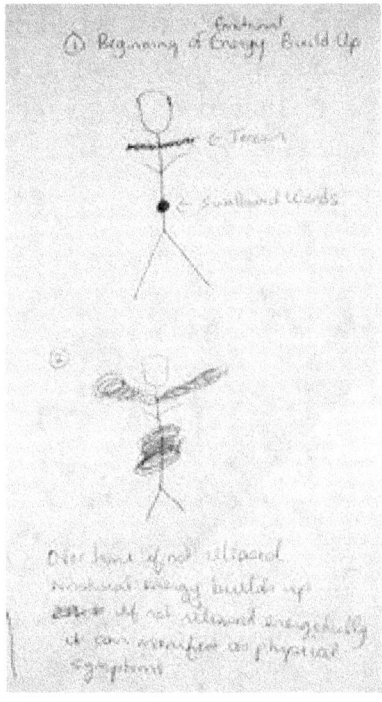

Please don't mistake these diagrams and words as me saying that stuck or old emotional energy is bad. It's an energy that can be transformed.

"All emotions are equal, welcome, and valid."

Patricia Clum

As old energy, emotions, and patterns are lifted using the techniques in this book, know that the release can happen slowly and gently, or quickly and fiercely. There are many ways to release energy. There is no right way and everyone is different.

"*Feeling is Healing.*"

I love the story I saw many years ago of a culture (where exactly I do not remember, perhaps Italy), where when a person in the community dies the women wail and cry and bang their fists on the coffin as part of the grieving process. It shocked me at first but I thought how important it is to release emotions physically during their natural rising!

Before I share more to help you feel and release buried emotions, I want you to know you can still be a good little child, an upstanding adult, a citizen of the world, while fully experiencing and moving all your emotions. You have the potential to be your best self when you allow full emotional expression. It creates space for more life to flow through you when you are fully present to your wholeness. (Keeping certain appropriateness in mind. It may or may not be best to let a fit of anger out in the grocery store for example.)

Participate fully in your emotional expression! A good place to start if you feel out of touch and you think there is something buried that is holding you back is to begin writing. You can start with "I invite myself to feel all of my feelings" or even "I don't know what to write".

You can write about what you are noticing. How does your body feel, what is happening in your life, what do you desire?

Write to your body.

Write to an emotion.

Write to or about another person.

Write to an area of your life you have a heavy experience with such as food, work, chores, technology, or money. Whatever comes up is excellent. Write and breathe and write until you can't write anymore. I've written one line to fully express, and I've scrawled forty pages to get to the depth of an emotion wanting to come out through physical expression.

Two practical ways to begin to get trapped or stagnant energy to move is through vocal expression and bodily movement. Physical and vocal expression are transformative energy mastery tools. This can feel super awkward at first but it is very impactful when you get into it. If you have a primal scream deep inside but you're not ready to let it out, just start making noises. I like to grunt and growl to start the flow of vocal expression when I'm releasing anger. Grrrrrr.

Loud sighing is great. Ooo. Aaaaaahhhhhhhh.......

I like to move my body along with the grunts and growls and sighs. Swaying, shaking my limbs, stomping. Getting in touch with anything deeper that wants to be expressed. Working my way to a scream or howl if there is one. The car is a great safe place to let the loud expressions out. There's nothing quite like screaming at the top of your lungs and saying all you need to say while driving (keeping your eyes on the road and hands on the wheel of course).

Years ago, I was getting in touch with my authentic self and releasing all the layers of masks and buried emotions that kept me from expressing myself for decades before. During this time, for about three months, a few times a week while driving to a friend's I would spend the twenty-minute drive yelling, screaming, and letting old words out I had never spoken. Honestly, a few times I wondered if I was going crazy but had great teachers in my life encouraging me to release and so I did! Gradually, the need to let these old words and energy out of my system slowed, and I had no more need to release in this way. A great teacher of mine, Patricia Clum summed it up nicely when she shared her wisdom, "a thousand years, a thousand tears." This was in reference to her own experience of having to cry for what seemed like months.

On the path of energy mastery, it's not about controlling your emotions but about letting them move through you. When you've suppressed them for so long, sometimes unknowingly, they will come up. I invite you to let them move, feel them fully, knowing they are not who you are, and as they move you create more space for truth and beauty in your life.

I feel comfortable enough with my full expression now that if I feel the need I can come home from my day, close my office door, and scream into a pillow two or three times. It's amazing how emotional release can reset the nervous system! Your nervous system loves movement, dancing, laughter, and breathing. It is how energy is conducted through your body. It is affected by your posture and governs empathy and feeling your environment.

All of you is magnificent. All of you is more than ok. More depth and love live underneath all your emotional expression. Keep your energy and emotions flowing. Find a safe place to let go. Reach out for help when you need it and never stop growing.

As you let go of old ideas that certain emotions are "bad" and fully express yourself, clear your energy, and step into your power, you will need some tools to protect your energy so you can maintain your new clarity and inner freedom. These tools are not meant to cut you off from other people. They are to give you space to truly strengthen your inner connection. Over time you can drop all of your protection and survival mechanisms when they aren't needed since there is no real danger. Through discernment, both mental and energetic, you integrate the meaning of:

> "*Do not cast your pearls before swine.*"
>
> Matthew 7:6

This means you can be true to yourself and share with those who are on the same path or curious about it. You don't share or only share what is necessary with those who are critical or judgmental. Some folks simply aren't interested in spirituality or even nutrition and they may be critical or make jokes about the topics when they are brought up. I have become both discerning enough to not bring the topics up around those who are this way or to bring it up in a way they can relate to. Often simply accepting the other person for who and where they are is enough to open them up. This keeps me in integrity and my power. I know that all I can do in these situations is to continue to work at being my best which may or may not be an example for others. The idea is to be aware of your energy and the energy of others so you stay aligned with yourself and prevent future issues of being entangled with others in ways that serve neither of you.

> *"In addition to all this, take up the shield of faith, with which you can extinguish all the flaming arrows of the evil one. Take the helmet of salvation and the sword of the Spirit, which is the word of God."*
>
> Ephesians 6: 16-18

Knowing how to shield and clear your energy can be incredibly useful tools at the beginning of your energy mastery journey, and ones you can take with you into the future.

The following are some of my favorite tools to protect and maintain your energy:

*Shielding and Bubbles of Light

To put up a shield is simple. You say "Shield" or ask for a shield to be placed around you. It may be helpful to visualize the color of the shield. You can also ask to be shown what color your shield is and listen for the answer, whether you hear or see it. For example, if you ask "show me my shield", and in your mind's eye you see a pink shield, then you know moving forward you can call on your pink shield at any time.

Another way of seeing this is by visualizing yourself wrapped in a bubble of protective loving energy. Shields or bubbles of light are helpful when going out into large crowds where there are many different types of people with many different intentions. This is a particularly useful tool for empaths at the beginning of their journey. It allows you to maintain an external boundary while you maintain and nurture your inner connection with your true self.

*The Zip Up

This quick tool is used to close energy leaks. Simply asking for energy leaks to be plugged can work in a pinch. An energy healing practitioner can help with this, or a simple tool to do with yourself is the zip up. Starting at the base of your spine visualize and make the action of doing up a zipper, slowly, all the way to the top of your head. This motion both gives you a little energy boost and closes off any leaks. Learning to close leaks in all areas of life over time will help you become aligned with your soul force. The more integrity you are living in, the more power you have to overcome obstacles in your life.

*Keep only what is yours.

This tool is great if you are suddenly feeling drained or not right. If this happens you can ask what is not yours to leave. Sometimes through life, you can pick up others' energies, and if you aren't diligent about your energy mastery they can stay with you for hours, days, or even longer. This is why the inner connection is so crucial. To do this, simply ask what's not yours to leave, and notice how you feel. This simple request can assist in learning from the past. If you notice anything leaving and you suddenly feel better, you may have a flash of insight as to where it came from, and that teaches you how not to get into the same situation again, perhaps by using a shield or bubble of light in those situations.

It's not always easy to keep your energy clear but these simple tools can help. I remember working in a retail natural health grocer and having to talk to a hundred people a day about their health, I am pretty good at keeping my energy clear but I also learned a ton about myself and how to maintain my inner connection with all sorts of people and situations. Each of these tools, but specifically this one helped immensely.

*Cutting cords

Sometimes you need to cut cords that have developed between yourself and others. Over the years of working with people, one of the most common energetic patterns that hold people in the past is energetic "cords" connecting the client with someone from their past. Often it is an old partner, an ex-boyfriend, or girlfriend, but it can also be a parent, grandparent, even a teacher, coach, or mentor. As you spend more and more time with one individual you develop bonds, which at the moment are generally good, but when the relationship breaks down or the connection fades, or a person passes, these cords can keep people stuck even though they are aching to move forward with their lives.

Science is now proving that you share energy with others. You may know this intuitively as you feel "connected to others" or you feel the energy of peoples and places. The connection isn't the problem at the moment, it's the lasting entanglements that prevent current energy flow. I've witnessed people come to me for various reasons who have one cord, multiple cords, or even layered cords! Once cords are released with love and intention you can receive an incredible amount of fresh energy to let go of the drain of what isn't serving you. Then, with this new energy, you are free to create in new ways you could not previously perceive.

How do you cut cords? Again, simply asking can be enough. Who are you asking? It could be your highest self, the Divine or God of your understanding, or Heavenly Angels. In my work when there are cords and entanglements I call on Archangel Michael to assist. This Archangel works on behalf of the Divine and has a mighty sword for cutting cords swiftly and gracefully.

Use your intentions to clear your energy and cut cords. This can be done daily if you work with lots of people, or once in a while if you've developed a connection that you feel is blocking you from taking your next steps. This can even be done in loving long-term relationships. In this case, it's not about severing the bond, but about maintaining your authentic voice in a healthy interdependent relationship. This is especially important when one person in the relationship needs to grow or is spiritually inclined and the other is not, perhaps they are settled and happy and not interested in spiritual things or making changes in their life. These are both ok, but if the spiritually inclined person is feeling out of sorts, asking for cords that do not serve to be cut and cleared can help maintain, reset, and raise spiritual energy.

I was once in a wonderful, connected relationship with a lovely man, yet once in a while, I would settle in while my soul was calling me to my deeper spiritual work. He was supportive of it, but he wasn't interested in doing the work himself. I fully accepted this and loved him anyway. Once in a while when I had to get down to business I would do a cord-cutting and energy clearing, placing him and myself in separate bubbles of light, asking for cords to be removed, and calling on my soul to be fully present so I could do my work. This allowed me space to complete a project I was working on AND bring my full self to the relationship.

Take a moment to contemplate if there are any cords in your life from current experience or past relationships that can be cut. If you find one, ask for it to be cut, breathe deeply, and notice how you feel.

One final note on protecting yourself is you don't do it from a place of fear or being spiritually mightier than others. You do it from a place of love, first for yourself, and then for others. You do it from a place of your truth and connection with the Divine so you can shine more in the world. You do it from a place of moving toward your goals. If you are constantly letting others bring you down it is hard to focus on where you are going. Where you are going might be an external destination but I also mean the deepening inner connection with the Divine that you are called to display in everyday life.

Other tools of note:

I will also briefly mention various other tools that I am not currently an expert in but when I have experienced them they are effective. If the information I mention resonates with you please follow your guidance and do your research and have your own experience with it. The tools of Neuro-Linguistic Programming (NLP) and the Emotional Freedom Technique (EFT) have been great tools for me that I encourage you to try for yourself.

NLP is a form of psychology, communication, and an approach to personal development that focuses on how words and phrases affect us at the internal level which then reflects into the outer world.

I first heard of NLP while doing Tony Robbins' Personal Power program in 2015. At the time I didn't know what it meant but I learned so much that I developed a respect for NLP even though I wasn't sure what it was. It wasn't until 2019 when I became a certified Neuro-Linguistic Programming Practitioner that I understood its effectiveness in life. NLP is a skill set that can be developed by anyone and if you feel a curiosity about it, especially if talking about energy seems too woo-woo for you, you may thrive using NLP's techniques.

Emotional Freedom Technique/Tapping-
EFT is a simple tool to release trapped energy and emotion and helps you get out of your head when you are nervous. You can see many guided videos on EFT on the internet for all sorts of topics.

EFT, also known as "tapping", is world-renowned for helping victims of trauma rebalance their nervous system and release fear. I have used EFT when working through strong emotions to help them clear faster, and when going to events where I was nervous about the crowd and before speaking engagements where I would be sharing something deeply personal. Before doing the tapping sequences I was nervous and anxious, and after I felt calm and relaxed to network and deliver my talk with ease. I no longer worried about what anyone else thought about me because I was centered in my heart and rooted in my power.

Exercise, Yoga, Intuitive movement, and Stretching to move energy.

Even if you don't know anything about yoga or another style of exercise go with your gut and what fits your schedule. I find yoga useful specifically because we often store emotions in our body and practices such as Yin Yoga, where you hold the poses for extended periods, help to release these emotions through movement and breath. It's potent stuff!

In 2009 I went to my first yin yoga class. As I relaxed into the poses, feelings, and emotions of all sorts arose and released through sustained stretching and deep breathing guided by an excellent teacher. In the final pose, we had our backs on yoga blocks, allowing our hearts to be stretched wide open to the sky. Before this moment, I had never known the true beauty of my own heart. I left the class feeling freer than I had in a long time.

You don't need to go out and learn all of the tools and modalities to master your energy but if you read this book and implement everything to the best of your ability you will be ten thousand times more proficient than someone who only reads and does not implement. This chapter has offered multiple tools you can add to your energy mastery toolbox.

In the next chapter, you will learn tools to overcome obstacles as they come up so you reach your goals. These tools will help you with obstacles of all sizes, from what seem like insurmountable mountains, to tiny bumps that lead to procrastination and feelings of helplessness. Read on...

Chapter 9

Take Action

You must have a great attitude in life. There will be days when you will want to whine and complain but you must not let this attitude rule. How do you know if you have a good attitude? You always (as much as possible) focus on the positive, put on your rose-colored fun glasses, and feel gratitude. You surround yourself with high vibe positive people who don't want to sit around commiserating. It's ok to share your challenges and seek support, of course, but if you make a habit of focusing on your problems you will stay in the same place.

I vividly remember one of my clients at the bank where I used to work who always seemed a little flustered describing me as "awfully optimistic". I smiled and wondered to myself, "what is so awful about being optimistic?" I know for sure I'd rather be optimistic than pessimistic. I've been in both places and optimism is way more fun and a better feeling place to be!

When you focus on the positive it's like keeping the doors to possibility open. No one wants to work with a negative person so... be a positive person! Bring joy wherever you go! Joy is who you truly are after all. If someone is telling you all the bad things in their life, or you are focused there yourself, simply ask "tell me something positive" or "ok thank you for sharing, now tell me some good news". This isn't to be rude or dismissive of other people's real issues or not having empathy, but as mentioned before, it can be easy to get stuck. Remaining aware and focusing on the positive is an absolute must!

Be a pollyanna.
Pollyanna: A person characterized by irrepressible optimism and a tendency to find good in everything. (Merriam Webster)

If you want to master your energy, and you do, you must make yourself see the bright side of life. You are a whole being and life is made up of the positive and negative yes, but what you focus on expands. When you focus on the positive in life it naturally keeps you motivated and moving forward. Positive is an open-hearted stance towards life. Negative is a closed-hearted stance towards life.

No one likes a "Debbie Downer" so be positive! (No offense if your name is Debbie, I use that slang term based on a popular Saturday Night Live sketch to make a point.) Even when you don't feel like it, you can start to build a new habit of looking on the bright side. Even if you are at a low point in your life or stuck in a rut you can rest assured that "this too shall pass". Habits are crucial to overcoming obstacles. Seeming obstacles can always be broken down through good habits, perseverance, dedication, and consistency. You currently have a whole slew of habits, both good and bad which you can review and determine if they are supportive of your dreams or not. Habits, whether they are good or bad are hard to break so obviously you want to have more good habits than bad.

To break old habits you must begin with the awareness that you are doing the habit, whether this is after you've done the thing, or during the doing of it, or as you are about to do the thing you no longer wish to do. Notice, and notice again next time, and over time begin to interrupt the pattern by doing something extravagant or extreme.

Let's say you have a habit of overeating at night that you wish to change. Notice when you are looking in the fridge for something to eat and then say out loud 'I am choosing health" as you slam the door and then go work on a project you've been saying you would do for years.

It's amazing how much time you waste doing bad habits when you say you want to do all these other things. Building new habits takes time and dedication. You have pathways built in your brain to the old ways of being so new inroads must be built!

Changing habits can be frustrating both mentally and emotionally as you go through it because you are changing your brain's neural pathways. Choose your habits wisely, they will impact your entire life and once they are built they are hard to break. In the beginning, new habits can seem hard to sustain but return again and again to your goal and the new habit you want to build until it is ingrained in your brain. Eventually, it becomes easy, like second nature.

I had to build new habits to write this book. I don't particularly enjoy writing and have had a massive amount of resistance to the idea of "discipline" my entire life but my higher self calls me to it. Now, I have cultivated the habit of surrender to the divine calling on my heart, which allows me to implement new habits that support me on my path.

To write this book I implemented a system where I would write first thing in the morning. I wake up, make myself my single cup of coffee for the day, and write while drinking it. I learned from my friend Gerry Roberts that you can write your book in a few minutes at a time, so that's how I began. When you sit for five minutes it easily turns into twenty when you can find a flow. For me, if I tried to set a goal of writing for an hour every day I would harbor resistance and resentment and probably never sit down to write or I would only do it once a month with great struggle. By starting slow, which you can with any new habit, and implementing five minutes a day I wrote the basis of my book in three months and have a new habit of content creation with which I can use to uplift those I serve.

What habits are you choosing?
Decide now which new habits you will build and which ones you will let go of.
Write them in your journal and go for it!

New Habits I am Building:

Old Habits I am Releasing:

If you need help get it by reaching out to my team or finding a qualified coach or behavioral therapist. You have an incredible amount of habits and when you become aware of them you can forge ahead creating new ones that create the lasting positive change you want to see in yourself.

"Be the change you wish to see in the world."

Mahatma Gandhi

~Goals~

Goals are truly important in energy mastery. Without goals, well, you get where you are going.

No goals = no direction = no particular destination.

Goals = direction = desired destination.

When you have a goal and you've mastered your energy you can use both of these factors to check in with yourself and measure your progress. You must be in alignment with your goals to make them happen. For example, you cannot continue to be lazy and eat junk food and expect to feel fabulous and fit. If you set a goal to feel fabulous and fit and then define some of the terms that let you know when you've achieved it, such as a certain weight, feeling, having a green smoothie every day, etc. You can begin to align your actions with your desired results. While you may not feel fabulous and fit in the beginning stages, you can measure your progress and notice how much more fabulous and fit you feel with each passing day. This can encourage you and create positive reinforcement to continually take the specific actions that align with your goal.

Your goals and intentions have to be laser sharp.

> *"Turn your shoulds into musts."*
>
> Tony Robbins

You can start with small goals to help build trust in yourself, then build momentum. Ultimately you:

> *"Gotta aim high cause life's what you make it."*
>
> The New Electric

When it comes to going for your goals it's important to have a supportive network whether it's a circle of friends who support you or a coach who guides you and kicks your ass when you need it.

Boundaries are also important for reaching your goals. Without boundaries, you might be willing to step over your desired actions, which can spiral into more of the same, like stashing your passion project in the closet or skipping a workout. If you miss your actions once in a while that's one thing, but if you continually fall out of step with your action plan then you are doomed for "failure" and lack of true fulfillment. If you never really go for your goals you may want to re-evaluate and see if those goals are actually what you want, need, and desire for yourself. Your goals should be true from your heart and call you forward, not something you think you should want.

"Actions make miracles."

The Luminaries

One of the most effective ways to overcome obstacles and stay on track to reach your goals and dreams is to get some accountability.

Accountability: the quality of being accountable or responsible; an obligation or willingness to accept responsibility or to account for one's actions. (Merriam Webster)

You can be accountable to yourself as you grow in maturity and find inner alignment with your goals.

However, what is most effective is having an accountability partner. Someone to hold you to it, motivate you when you don't feel like it, give you tools to help you succeed, and someone to share your wins with. A good accountability partner, whether it's a good friend, a like-minded group, or someone you pay like a coach, will reflect your goals and greatness back to you. They will hold you to the higher standard you have set for yourself.

Great accountability partners don't take your B.S. They call out your magnificence when you can't see it, and they love you through the challenges and help you find the way through. If you've never worked with a coach or mentor before and are curious about what it can do for you, book your Energy Coaching call with me at www.VickiAdrianne.com.

Having a team, whether it be you and another, or a group, is incredibly effective at helping you break through obstacles. The reason is these other people, if they are qualified, high-quality individuals, can see your blind spots and help you maneuver so those spots are covered and don't take you down in moments when you are nearing a breakthrough.

A way to discover your blind spots or to help another discover theirs is to ask,
"What do I think might get in the way of doing the thing (taking the action, saying the thing, getting the goal)?

When you take genuine space and time to answer this question you may see some things in a new light.

Having a team supporting you allows you to receive feedback and suggestions for continual growth. They can call you out on your own stories holding you back. They can hold you accountable when you are teetering on the edge of giving up. They can celebrate you every step of the way regardless of whether they are celebrating getting out of bed for the day after a major setback, or celebrating the launch of a passion project that has taken you years to launch. Having a team is not only supportive but makes life as a whole more enjoyable. You are not meant to go through this life alone!

~Beware the lizard brain!~

A major factor that holds humans back from overcoming seeming obstacles is your "lizard" brain or survival mechanism which wants to keep you safe and small. This part of us has indeed kept us safe and allowed us to evolve this far, but it is not equipped for the rapid pace of technological and other industrial and political growth of the past century.

This part of you would have you seek comfort when your heart is calling out for adventure, risk, and ultimate growth. This part of you can sabotage your best efforts to go after your dreams if you are not aware of it. This part of you can be wily, so it's important to become aware of how it operates in your life.

Take a moment to journal what thoughts or behaviors come up when you want to get out of your comfort zone.

Here are some questions to help suss out what your lizard brain's survival mechanism might be:

♥ What happens for you when you feel "unsafe", (whether you are actually safe or not)?

♥ What is your pattern of action or way of being when you are working on a breakthrough but something is holding you back?

♥ What is it that continually keeps you stuck?

These may be easy to answer or require some soul searching. As I said, it's sneaky. The job of this part of you is to protect you and it's primal. Thankfully you are now in a place in time where you can become aware of it and open to higher consciousness.

Naming your survival mechanism can help you call it in with love and non-judgment which is crucial for all true transformation. Taking the time to listen to what a part of you needs loosens the grip it has on you. Your survival mechanism can be like a small child fearfully gripping its parent's legs, not letting go, and making it difficult for the adult to move. Once the child realizes it is safe and receives the love and attention it needs, it loosens his grip and returns to his normal pace of life.

Here are a few examples;

-You want to try something new but your habit is to revert to doing what the "responsible" thing is such as cleaning the house, reviewing current financials, or trying to control a certain situation or outcome. You might call this one Responsible Ruth/Rudy.

-You live with others who are not in the same boat but YOU want to reach a fitness goal such as running a five or ten-kilometer run, or a half or full marathon, but when you think of it instead of putting your sneakers on you suddenly feel tired and need to take a nap or get cozy on the couch to watch t.v. with the others. You can call this one Lazy Lucy/Lui.

This part of you may be protecting your relationships with loved ones, but holding you back from reaching your own goals. If you truly want to reach a goal but don't listen and take action, your relationships will eventually be strained as you are not being true to yourself. In these circumstances energy mastery and a strong communication channel are vital. When you can speak your truth and go for what you want, you can maintain harmony in your home even if you and your loved ones have different goals.

By the way, good relationships are the foundation of all abundance in life. And all relationships are a mirror of your relationship with yourself.

"To thine own self be true."

Polonius in Hamlet by Shakespeare

-You want to speak up more or be seen in your true light and try something new but every time you go to do the thing that will make the difference you doubt yourself and shrink back. Perhaps you numb yourself with t.v., food, or hiding in your room, perhaps even reading a personal development book or taking a course in the name of "getting better". You can call this one Scaredy Cat Sally/Sam.

-You want to invest in a new course/program/education, outfit/stylist, personal trainer or coach, or even take a dream trip but you hold back saying you can't afford to invest in yourself. You can call this one Broke Becky/Bob.

The survival mechanism is strong and sneaky. Now that you have this awareness notice what takes you out, or where you hold back and give this part of you a name. Call it into your awareness fully, lovingly. Ask it what it needs. Perhaps you need to take a day off so you can feel rested to get out there, perhaps you need to start a savings plan and still invest in yourself. Listen listen listen and nurture all of you so you can have space to truly go for it. If you ignore these parts or lack awareness of them they can take over and then you wonder why you aren't making changes you want to see/be.

Your daily musts for overcoming obstacles are:

- Living with intention. Think about and then consciously set intentions for how you want to feel, be, express yourself, and create on this day.
- Choose your highest potential., You are always able to make a conscious choice. You get to choose how to act, how to respond to situations. You get to choose to continue to move forward even in the face of obstacles. You can choose to honor yourself. Choose to say yes or no. Choose to ask for help. If you feel stuck, make a deliberate choice, and act from there.

Remember that it is necessary to have a vision.

"Where there is no vision, the people perish."

Proverbs 29:18

Vision boards are worthwhile since they constantly remind you of where you are going. Now there is a truth about vision boards that hasn't been talked about much and it is that they are truly meant to be representations of the inside of you. They are not about creating anything from outside of yourself because well, frankly that is impossible. All creativity comes from within. The Law of Attraction isn't about being in lack and trying to magnetize what you don't have. It is about harmonizing within so your inner peace generates more happiness and freedom and alignment from this place which then draws more of those conditions to you.

Vision boards themselves aren't the problem, vision boards are amazing. I strongly urge you to create a vision board as a representation of what is on the inside of you, your vision, not just material things you want. When you create it this way, you already have access to your vision as it lives within you, and having a physical vision board helps keep you in alignment. When you look at it you want to feel your success, feel your alignment with what you already have access to within, and are now creating.

Feel your way day by day, step by step, always being true to your heart's vision.

Many years ago, as I opened up to my purpose I received a vision of myself on stage speaking on the topic of empowerment to a large group of women. At the time I had almost zero public speaking experience save the speech writing class in grade six and some presentations in my university days. I felt this vision so forcefully within me that within the next three months my heart led me to take a speaker development mastermind program. I created my vision board and had no idea how the vision would manifest but I stayed true to my heart. When the opportunity presented itself to speak at the Fearless Women's Summit in Halifax, Nova Scotia in front of a delegation of 650 women I knew this was the manifestation of my vision! I still had tons of work to do and when I finally stepped on stage the energy and knowing that this was exactly what I had seen in my vision four years prior was visceral!

You will notice my vision board doesn't even have a picture of me on stage as you might expect of a vision board. What you do see is a representation of what I needed to become. I needed to feel beautiful and safe being seen. I needed to feel confident truly expressing myself and I needed to promote myself as a speaker to get the gig. Creating a vision board can be a mystical experience of tapping into truth and asking to be shown what is needed on the vision board. This is what I created and as I reflected on it daily I was guided to take the actions that led to becoming all I needed to fulfill the vision!

When you are in alignment with your true goals your heart won't let you give up. True goals are the key here. This is the secret to fulfilling your dreams and never giving up. True goals and life purpose pathways are different for everyone and I stress this point because for some it may be about material goods and that's ok. What I find most people do is think material goods are their true goals when in fact their authentic goals are about embodying their creativity and self-expression fully. And how this manifests is unique to everyone.

When you've got your vision and your heart is open you can take steps day after day towards becoming that vision. You try many different things and learn from each step. Perhaps you take a break if you are feeling temporarily stuck and have some fun to gain new inspiration. Then try again from new angles and using different methods.

You cannot fail when you don't give up.

Side note, you can never really plan or be fully prepared for what will show up in life. That is the joy of this glorious divine mystery. But you can plan and prepare to the best of your ability, continue to have goals to reach, and use the tools in this book to address and grow through all of life's captivating lessons. Never stop learning, stay curious and connected to your center, and never give up.

And truth be told, if you have the vision, you have the means to create it. There is no separation and the creation of your vision is the most wonderful adventure you can embark on.

You may be thinking "but what if I am, or I become, really stuck. Like, *really* stuck?"

If you ever find yourself in this place, relax and breathe. Your ability to get some elevation and take the birds-eye view can help you move forward. To get the birds-eye view take a moment to shake off any frustration or tiredness you are feeling. I mean really shake! Get up, shake your arms and your legs, wiggle your hips, move your energy! Give yourself a true break where you don't have to think about your current situation or how you are going to achieve your vision. Let go, just for a moment. This may require going for a walk in nature to take in earth's beauty. Bring your journal into nature with you, or wait until you get home and begin by reflecting on where you are today, where you began, and where you are going. Keep your mind open to allow the bigger picture to be seen.

A prompt to get even more clarity and insight is to ask "What am I missing?" or "What do I need to surrender so I can let go of what is blocking me?" Let the answers flow. This exercise allows you to take a step back without disengaging completely and sabotaging your progress.

"Surrender" is an act of letting undeniable love and forgiveness into your life and choosing to stay true to your heart as it unfolds. The practice of divine surrender has given me a sense of peace that has never left me, whether I am feeling "stuck" or completely aligned in action.

We've already talked about meditation but it might surprise you to know that meditation, even though it is a still quiet practice, is amazing at helping you break through barriers and obstacles. Sitting quietly and observing your breath and allowing your thoughts to pass by without interfering or attaching resets your focus to what you would like to be focusing on. When you meditate you create space for new energy and ideas that can be the inspiration you need to move forward. You've probably heard about how the best ideas come when you are in the shower? This is because your mind isn't overthinking which allows space for new ideas and energy to come in. I get my best insights while walking in the forest.

Meditation refreshes your body and mind and can allow you to gain insight into the root of what may be holding you back. For example, limiting beliefs or past experiences. If you are feeling stuck, you can enter into meditation to uncover what is going on. Simply acknowledge you are feeling blocked and ask for the root of the block to be revealed.

This is also a great exercise if you are feeling triggered by something or someone outside of yourself. In this case, ask to be shown the root of why you are feeling or reacting this way. I've used this many times in my life when I overreacted to something. One time many years ago I had a crush on a man who lived in another country and sent him a "Happy Thanksgiving" message on his country's day of celebrating this holiday.

His response was a simple "Thank you, I appreciate you."

As simple as this was it sent me into intense reactionary upset. I felt angry, hurt, and sad and I didn't know why! To help myself through my reaction I entered into meditation and asked for inner guidance. "Why is this upsetting me?"

What was revealed made total sense! I had heard those words "I appreciate you" from another man with whom things did not work out well which had left an impression on my subconscious that a man could appreciate me and still hurt me deeply. There had been an internal connection there which created a distrust of men that was being shown to me through my reaction.

The answer didn't come immediately. I had to sit with the discomfort for about five minutes before the unconscious could be made conscious and the wait was worth it. I was then able to offer some forgiveness and healing to myself and others and claim my power back while declaring and intending new beliefs about being able to trust again.

When you can be patient, get some elevation on your place and perceptions in life, and do some internal excavating you reveal and heal all that no longer serves you. This allows you to continue to move forward in glory and grace.

If you are feeling stuck and on a deadline here is how to bust through seeming obstacles in five minutes or less; get out some paper or your journal and write out all your fears and frustrations in the current moment.

Specifically as related to your obstacle but also include anything else on your mind.

Write what you are afraid of. What do you think will happen if you take the step? What will happen if you don't? Once you get that all out, write what you are making all of this mean about you.

Make sure you get all of your emotions out onto the paper. If there are any left you may not be able to move forward. This writing exercise can end up being one paragraph, or fifteen pages, it doesn't matter as long as you get it out! You will know when you are done writing because suddenly you will feel free to do the task you were having a hard time getting into. You may even free flow out a solution to your current obstacle or problem through the writing process or think of new creative ways to do what you are wanting to do!

I've used this tool many times to get out my fears and frustrations about doing a task. It always reveals some limiting belief or fear that, once down on paper, seems small and insignificant compared to the power and truth of who I am. Whereas when they are in my head and my energy field they are enough to take me off my purposeful track.

You may find that the more you do this exercise the less you have to do it because you are getting everything out that stands in the way of achieving your goals. If you come across something such as a habit, thought, experience, or pattern that continues to show up simply notice it. When you have the time, dive into it a little bit deeper in meditation, journaling, or working with a coach to unravel its hold in your life and build new habits that support your goal. Decide that you have the power to create what you desire!

These activities help you become and maintain integrity in your life. If you say you want to create something but you continually put it off due to how you are feeling or other obstacles, your heart knows and over time this can become an energy clouding over your heart's voice and truth.

Integrity is defined as the state of being whole or undivided. Living in integrity means doing what you say you will do, and living your values and ideal beliefs from the inside out. As you master your energy, anywhere you are out of integrity will become a point of heightened awareness for you. This is an opportunity to move through the challenge, and integrate the lesson as part of your wholeness.

A desire to live in integrity is probably one of the greatest goals you can have at the beginning of your journey if you are currently out of integrity. In my own life, integrity had to come first before any of my other goals and dreams would manifest. If you are not in integrity you are sending mixed messages to the universe. You say you are or want one thing but act and feel another way- it's contradictory. It can create a lot of disillusionment and anger if you don't own your part in integral living. Integrity is being true to your highest calling.

Once truly set in place in your life, integrity is like a shield against wrongdoing or being. You begin to align on the inside with your goals, so doing anything out of alignment becomes a point of contraction you are no longer willing to put up with. In terms of energy mastery, it is a simple fact that you feel best and radiate the most light when you are in alignment with your inherent, natural goodness. Living in integrity keeps you rooted in truth which leads to great success and fulfillment in your life over the long term.

In 2011, at rock bottom after giving all of my power away, I dedicated my life to truth. This led to a series of events that helped my understanding of the importance of integrity. Being dedicated to living in truth meant I could no longer lie, cheat, or steal from others or myself. I had bad habits and ways of being that had to go and changing wasn't always easy. One by one, and sometimes all at once, I was shown where I was out of integrity which could be heart-wrenching and brought me to tears and sometimes to my knees in prayer to be helped through into my new, truth-based way of life.

My stake in the ground moment where I decided I needed to make a change and get clear on my purpose for life came from my rock bottom but yours doesn't have to. You can have a stake in the ground moment anytime you decide. Often these moments are brought about by crises, those times when you are so down and out that something needs to change. Even if you have been thinking of making a change or creating something different in your life, but you are currently comfortable and there doesn't seem to be any rush, you can still make a bold new declaration, your stake in the ground, of what you will create.

To make your stake in the ground moment the most impactful it can be helpful to think about and feel into all the reasons why what you are currently doing isn't working. On the flip side, think about why creating what you want will be good for you and the world. Once you are in your frustration of what isn't working, or the power of what you want to create, make a fierce action like you have a stake in your hand and you are putting it in the ground claiming your territory.

Put all of your energy and focus into this moment. As you are doing this make a **BOLD** declaration about what you are now standing for, that you are owning your power and doing what it takes to step into it. This could be about truly taking care of yourself (no more late-night junk food binges, implementing new health practices, etc.), or whatever you desire to claim in your life.

Now that you have put your stake in the ground and made your declaration you have created massive energy in the direction you want to go. Follow that energy forward. It may take you in unexpected directions. Pay attention and make sure you are opening up to greater alignment with your declaration. You may wish to use timelines or small goals if you have something specific you will work on. If you ever don't meet your deadlines, re-evaluate and make a new declaration from this point about how you will move forward. Don't beat yourself up about it.

Stake in the ground moments are not to be taken lightly. Most of the time, for most people, they aren't something consciously created. With solid intention and willingness to change you can create energy that opens new doors when you use this method of moving forward.

As you step into all that you are claiming and being and becoming in your life, it is imperative to be energetically empowered. This means you start with awareness and cultivate your energy to feel your best as much as possible. We all have down days and up days and everything in between, it's called being human. Energetic empowerment is about owning your yes and your no.

Energetic empowerment requires non-judgmental awareness of yourself, and embracing all that is with grace, and caring for yourself deeply. It involves having self-care practices rooted in your daily and weekly life. Being energetically empowered is allowing your emotions to fully express so they move through you and don't get stuck. It is about being and staying grounded while remaining connected to your open heart. It is caring for and loving others while helping them release their burdens without taking them on yourself.

Energetic empowerment is about being a channel, an open vessel for joy, grace, and love, and speaking your truth in all situations.

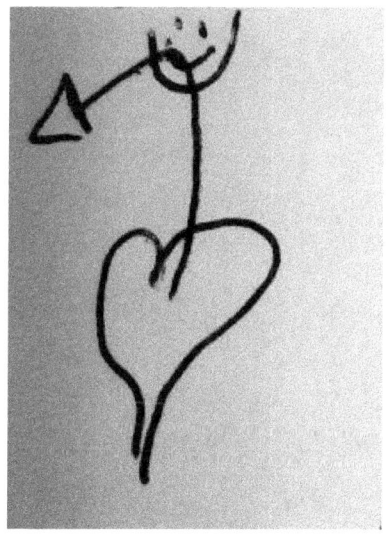

When you are energetically empowered you burst through obstacles. You shine and take action from the inside out. Nothing can stop you when you are aligned from within. If you are reading this book you will have everything you need to live a life of energetic empowerment and energy mastery.

Let me stress the importance of never giving up on yourself or your purpose and remember to put the inner voice of love and truth above all outer voices. In the next chapter, we will wrap it all up with the failsafe principle to get you through life in a way you love instead of just surviving.

Chapter 10

Never Give Up

"To know and not to do is not to know."

Confucius

Your attitude in life has the power to either close or open up possibilities! You've most likely heard the phrase "faith moves mountains" which is based on the Biblical story of Jesus' disciples not being able to help a man cure his son. After Jesus healed the son he said to his disciples;

"...Because you have so little faith. Truly I tell you, if you have faith as small as a mustard seed, you can say to this mountain, 'Move from here to there,' and it will move. Nothing will be impossible for you." -Matthew 17:20

Your attitude and results in life are a reflection of your faith. Whether your faith is in yourself, the divine, or whatever, you get to choose. I recommend a combination of your true self and the Divine which are never separate anyways. Having a positive attitude isn't about being a surface-level pollyanna, although it's a great start to raise awareness of what lies deeper within you. Having a great attitude is about having the inner conviction and knowing that life is good, you are joy, and if you've got the dreams and desire you can achieve it.

Your dreams are God's plan for your life.

When you live in a state of positivity and openness other people catch the energy and suddenly want to help you or point you towards something that could move you forward. Doors and windows open. You are shown where doors and windows close. While you may not understand why at the moment, you have faith and know it is what's best, and you can let it go and move forward in the direction you are being guided.

You have the attitude that you cannot fail unless you quit. Even if you quit temporarily, it doesn't last for more than a day or two as your inner drive moves you forward, naturally. You never truly give up because you have a vision, you trust yourself and have awareness of your inner guidance, and you have done the work to be in integrity with the truth that speaks from within.

Even if you have a bad day you know how to move the energy, not from a place of force, but through love and grace. You allow all emotions as part of your beingness in this human form. Yet you are rooted in joy and positivity. Over the long run, positivity makes everything better, and your acute awareness of anything lying beneath the surface gets handled in due time so you remain integral.

My dear friend Stacey Rae likens these things going on under the surface, or in the background, as the "pencil in the fan". They are only mildly annoying until you realize it is what is holding you back. When you become aware you can take action through many of the tools in this book, to remove the pencil from the fan, so you can flow forward.

For example, this could be a habit you have that is getting in the way of your greatness or a conversation you need to have that is on your mind, therefore, taking up space in your consciousness. It could be a thing you need to do that's long overdue and once you complete it, will create a whole new space within your being and environment to create massive growth.

Through all of the changes life brings, positivity lights the way from your heart, and forward through your journey. When you see the glass as not only half full but overflowing you are tapped into pure potentiality where you know you can create anything your true heart desires. Positivity can be the hope during a season or time of darkness. Not that you ignore the darkness or cover it over with pretend light, but hanging on to the knowing that "this too shall pass" and more joy will flow because it is who you are.

> *"Never give up. Never give up. Never Give up."*
>
> Winston Churchill

No one else is going to do your work for you. You must have a can-do attitude. Never giving up means never giving up, the same way "unconditional love" means unconditional. You may struggle and have strife, but you don't give up on your heart's true desires. I remember watching a video that enhanced my understanding of this. Hip-hop artist Snoop Dogg is giving a speech when he got his star on the Hollywood walk of fame. He thanks himself for all the hard work he put in, all the dedication he had, for believing in himself, for always being a giver, and for doing more right than wrong. Now you don't all have to be as famous or well-known as Snoop Dogg but you have something to offer when you are fully expressed in your true self as joy and love. This energy spreads and changes the world one breath at a time.

> *"It always seems impossible until it is done."*
>
> Nelson Mandela

When you think you "can't", remind yourself that you believe in yourself and you will find a way, even if that way is through surrender to the now. Start right where you are, always, and do what you can. The Law of Attraction is a real force in the Universe but you must be careful not to get stuck in spiritual bypassing. Spiritual bypassing is when you are telling yourself nice words and doing lots of "manifestation work" and expecting good returns without being in integrity and putting in the necessary outputs (actions) to truly bring those manifestations to you. It is listening for guidance and lining up your being with your doing to create more epic love in your experience.

A sure-fire way to make sure you are living successfully is to surround yourself with others who are working on their dreams too. Studies show that you are the average of the five people you spend the most time with. This is a call to be aware of your self-talk and how the behavior and words of others impact you. Are the people you spend the most time with bringing you down or encouraging a mindset of lack or inability to change? You may need to let them go, not by harshly cutting the relationship out, but slowly shifting to more positive relationships with others who are on the same growth and expansion path you are. You get to clarify your relationships so there is only room for positivity, honesty, and growth.

This is true for your environment as well. Your personal environment is a reflection of your consciousness. It also can impact your consciousness. Take a look around if you are at home, or think about your home and/or work environment and notice if it is messy, cluttered, is there any free space in the room for energy to flow?

When I talk about the environment I'm not only referring to the physical stuff either, I'm also referring to the energy of the room. You know how you can feel the energy of a space when you walk into it? How is the energy of your space? Does it make you feel peaceful, productive, frenzied, lazy, cramped, or expansive and creative?

I moved a lot in my twenties and early thirties so I became adept at clearing the energy of new spaces and setting the energy up for my continual growth and expansion. Here are some ways to clean the energy and set intentions for your space, as well as maintain the energy on an ongoing basis:

-Sit in the center of your room and imagine a vortex of energy swirling down through the center, like a bathtub draining. Imagine the energy getting cleansed as it is all brought down into the center of the earth. Next, turn the vortex into white light or your favorite color and slowly close off the vortex making sure every last bit of old energy is gone down through it, and then fill the space with white or colored light. Now set your intentions for the space. Breathe into your heart and ask the space to be filled with love, creativity, relaxation, productivity, whatever you would like your home to be space for.

-Set your favorite crystals around your home, on windowsills, or anywhere that feels right to you.

-Have Himalayan salt rock lamps in each room if possible, or wherever you spend most of your time. Salt rock lamps promote health by giving off negative ions that counteract the positive ions in the air which can make it hard to sleep.

-Burn sage or Palo Santo with intention to cleanse the energy.

-Use essential oils to support various moods, Frankincense is my favorite for clearing and setting new energy in a space. It reminds me of the idea of "holiness" or "wholeness", representing a way of being in divine service. Lavender is brilliant for helping you relax into a deep sleep.

-Use only all-natural cleaning and beauty products. If you are filling your home with toxic chemicals you may be harming your health and the health of the earth.

Now that we've covered your external environment, let's return to your internal environment. What is it like in there? Are you being kind to yourself? Do you have positive self-talk, appreciate your body, know your value, and believe you are worthy of the goodness of life? Do you believe you are smart and can figure anything out? Are you aware of your limiting beliefs and choosing to replace them with better, more supportive beliefs? Can you lift yourself up when you are down?

As a young woman, I was a terrible friend to myself. I truly hated my body and said all sorts of terrible things about myself every single day! This bled into my overall attitude about life and how it should/could/would be. Having "that's the way it is and I don't like it" beliefs is no way to move forward into energy mastery. Believing you can, and talking yourself through it, can seem like a lot of work in the beginning but it is worth it! You are worth it.

You can begin to own your right to lift yourself up. This will lead to naturally lifting others up as you identify with the truth of your love. Do you notice your self-talk? Notice over the next few days what you are saying to yourself and how your thoughts make you feel. As you become more aware you can shift your thinking. Some poor thoughts may still arise, that's normal, but you will become aware almost instantly as you have raised your standards. Then you can tell yourself that the negative thought isn't what is true, and then kindly but firmly remind yourself of the truth; you are (insert your favorite affirmation of truth here). For example, "I am love".

It's important to recognize when you are holding onto things from your past. We all do it, a lot of the time, and this is why self-forgiveness and the willingness and ability to let things go is a major skill set of energy mastery. Notice if you are holding past mis-takes over yourself. Mistakes are simply mis-takes and you can try again until you get it right. Are you holding any guilt or shame? It's time to let that go! As you master your energy and become all of who you truly are there isn't any room for that in your life. Do an inventory of your inner landscape, practice forgiveness as needed, and communicate openly with trusted advisors and loved ones.

There comes a point when the internal reference to Self as Love becomes so great that the outer work of expression and communication, regardless of how embarrassing or challenging it may feel at the time, becomes non-negotiable. You realize that you holding back is the only thing holding you back. You may feel that people think you are ridiculous or crazy, but as you grow and shine you may become an inspiration to them! Always choose to live as inspiration rather than in quiet internal desperation. Set yourself free.

One time during a retreat in San Diego, I realized at a profound level that wherever I felt held back by life, it was me holding myself back from life! The overarching intuitive message of the retreat for me was: 'It is all real; my truth and experiences are real and valid (I've been told I have an overactive imagination by people who don't believe in spiritual realms), and it's about to get a whole lot more real.'

As I opened my heart that day in San Diego I prayed for whatever was in me that kept me withholding from life be released, and to be shown a new way of being. I declared that life is too marvelous to hold myself back from all of it. As I move into this declaration I remain aware to look for and notice where I am holding myself back and do the work to stay open to love in all its forms and unfoldings.

As you let more and more go, through acts of forgiveness, it becomes clear you can be grateful for everything. Perhaps up to this point in your life, you have realized life's lessons are often the "refiner's fire". Your challenges help you focus on what is important and "burn away" what no longer serves you in the moment.

> *"There is divine purpose in the adversities we encounter every day.*
> *They prepare, they purge, they purify, and thus they bless."*

James E. Faust

Gratitude can help you turn your pain into passion. Notice if there is anything you are not grateful for and ask yourself what is it teaching you and see if you can find something to be grateful for. It helps to first practice gratitude for the things that are easy to be grateful for such as the roof over your head, the bed you sleep in, and the food you ate today.

When I got out of the situation where I gave my power away I was deeply in debt and afraid of the dark but I made a point every night and every morning to find things to be grateful for. It didn't seem like there was much at first! Many anxious nights and hopeful mornings in the beginning it was simple. "Thank you for the roof over my head, my bed, and the fact I got to eat today". I sincerely couldn't think of anything else but this practice was the catalyst to soon finding more things to be grateful for.

Now, many years later, I see how I can be grateful for just about everything in life. If there is something in my life that I am challenged by, I know and trust I will find a way to be grateful for it eventually. I savor the experience, feeling it all through an open heart to see how I can grow through it. Practicing gratitude when you are down has the natural effect of lifting you back up. If you can allow full acceptance and surrender to what is, it becomes easier to see the bigger picture through time. I invite you to begin noticing all you have to be grateful for, every day. If this seems too difficult currently I have a program designed to help you let go of what weighs you down so you can move on. You can learn more about Let Go and Live On on my website.

At your core, you are joy and love. It is up to you to cultivate this truth and create the state of being you want to live in. If joy is who you are, why not be it, and experience it as much as possible? To do this, you need to bring forth from within an enthusiasm for life. You get to be alive today! You get to be You today! How amazing is that!?

Enthusiasm is defined as intense excitement and comes from the Greek word "entheos" which means "possessed by God and inspired". Enthusiasm is a force that can change worlds. Nothing major ever got done without enthusiasm, even if it is quiet enthusiasm that delivers sustenance to move forward every day. I'm a big fan of boisterous enthusiasm because to me it feels fun, whether it's me giving it out or witnessing another in this state. How inspiring is it to see someone enthusiastically going for their dreams?

Focus on divine joy in all moments- knowing joy is your truth even in your lower energy moments. If you are feeling constricted, remember to breathe and stretch and allow your emotions to move through you. Never giving up requires having enthusiasm for living your truth, and you should be enthusiastic about that because in energy mastery there is no denying your truth. When you are in alignment with your truth you will know and it will guide you forward every day! The incredible thing about finding your truth is once you do, it is always there, and it continues to call more growth and evolution through you.

When you are on your path and never giving up it is important to celebrate! The scientific and spiritual fact that you are a miracle is enough to celebrate every day! When was the last time you truly celebrated yourself for all you have done in life or even a small thing you have accomplished or become?

A celebration is a formal recognition, acknowledgment, and ceremony of what you have done and who you have become. It is the action of marking one's pleasure at an important event or occasion by engaging in enjoyable, typically social, activity. (dictionary.com)

We often celebrate birthdays only intending to get together and eat cake and catch up. We sing a standard song and there may be gifts involved, but are you *truly* celebrating yourself, and all you have done on your last trip around the sun?

You don't have to wait for a birthday to celebrate either. If you can think of something you've accomplished recently that you haven't yet celebrated (I bet you can think of at least one thing) then have a little (or big) celebration. You can celebrate by having a dance party, taking a bath, getting a massage, going out for dinner, whatever you fancy. Be sure to bring the intention of celebrating! You deserve to be acknowledged. You are worth it and so much more.

When you celebrate it lets your subconscious mind know you've done this and come this far and are capable of much more. It completes a cycle and your mind loves completions! Completing cycles creates space for more energy of creation to flow so you have more to celebrate in the coming weeks, months, and years.

Celebrating only once a year on your birthday frankly is not enough. You are a miracle! Life is a miracle and you are out there every day doing incredible things, working through your healing, making moves, and creating waves. All of that deserves special acknowledgment through an act of celebration. We could all use more fun in our life so if you can add a splash of fun, excitement, or adventure to your celebration even better!

"Until further notice, celebrate everything."

Anonymous

Celebrating connects you with your divine self, and the ultimate goal in life is a purposeful expression of your divine self. When you realize this you can still have other, more specific goals but this larger purpose-based goal is one you can never forget. When you are on the path of living this goal, it is easy to be passionate about achieving it! Once you taste the truth of your heart and how good it feels to be fully expressed and continually unfolding, you won't want to give up or settle for less. The real goal is the inner drive of evolutionary expansion which continues forever- it simply won't allow you to give up on it. It is a natural force guiding you through life, helping you to continually become your best, whatever that is for you. This is true even when achieving the outcomes includes taking a nap.

Let the focus of your true goals be internal satisfaction, where peace reigns.

Remember that energy is everything. Have I mentioned the critical importance of positivity? I certainly know life can be the pits sometimes, but you always have access to move forward and choose where you focus your thoughts as you make your way through life's grand challenges. It is ok to feel down and experience all of your emotions, yes, yet your general disposition and outlook on life most of the time should be sunshine and expecting more sunshine. Positivity breeds positivity. Thinking on the bright side of life is a master habit that can be built. It is easy to slip into a negative state of mind if you are constantly surrounded by people with that outlook.

For example, you work with a group of people who think they are stuck in their jobs but they are doing it because they "have to" for the money, they hate Mondays and can never wait for the weekend. Be mindful to notice what they are saying and how they are behaving and choose your own better thoughts. You are there for a reason, even if you can't see it yet. You do your best and make time for all that you love. The job provides a certain lifestyle for which you are grateful, you get to help people every day. Whatever it is, be focused on the positive. Never let others bring you down. If they trigger you, use some of the tools mentioned in this book, and always stay open-hearted, connect to your inner joy, love, and peace, and know you are an ever-evolving being of love.

Take a breath, smile, and feel into your heart now. How grand is this connection? Many people walk through life only in their heads, completely disconnected from their hearts. While this is changing on a grand scale, still the majority of the population is disconnected from their source of joy. Be grateful that you are strongly connected and that you can spread this love outward.

~A note on "resting bitch face"~

I have resting bitch face, or RBF, an unpleasant term for people who look serious most of the time. I have already shared that I tend to take life too seriously and this is something I am successfully tackling to let joy and lightheartedness flow more easily in my life. One of the easiest things I have taken on is to smile more. Smile for no reason, smile when driving to work, heck I'm smiling while I write this because I have reminded myself of this simple life-brightening practice.

While it's true smiling takes fewer muscles than frowning, it has a profound effect on your physiology! Smiling for no reason may take a bit more effort, perhaps because you are fighting gravity by lifting your cheeks but doing so creates a chain reaction from your face into your whole body. When you smile you begin to feel lighter, you may appear more approachable (maybe that's just me, or if you tend to have resting bitch face you know what I mean). Smiling can make you think you have lots to smile about, and you do, you may have temporarily forgotten. Smiling isn't only an action for your face, but for your body and your soul too! Practice smiling and you will naturally smile more. Give it a try!

Laughter lets the light out.

In the way that smiling positively affects you, laughter is potent medicine for all the ills of life. Laughter is joy that cannot be contained. I love this quote I saw one day:

> *"How wonderful is it that we laugh because our bodies cannot contain the joy!"*

Unknown

Laughter can be natural or even forced or created. You may have heard of laughter yoga where you start laughing and it creates a ripple effect from there. You are joy at your center and when you connect with it through laughter the effects are undeniable. Laughing is an abdominal exercise that puts you in touch with your core. When you have a big belly laugh it forces all of the old air out of your lungs and brings in fresh oxygen, the best kind of deep breathing!

When was the last time you had a good laugh? For me, it was yesterday (it's early morning as I write this and I hope there is lots more laughter today!) Can you just be silly? I used to be so tightly wound up that being silly felt totally awkward! Now I'm ok with it because I am aware not to judge myself (most of the time, I'm human too and not perfect!) Go ahead and have a laughing fit! Invite others to join you, bring the joy that you are out into the world!

On the note of getting old air out of your lungs, this is another excellent practice that is simple yet profound. When you live your life only breathing into the top of your lungs via shallow breathing the air in the bottom of the lungs can get "stale". By doing a long slow inhale, followed by a fast and direct exhale, making sure to empty the lungs, you can then bring fresh air into the body. Get the old out and bring the new in whether it's through laughter or another practice you take on. It's another tool in your energy mastery toolbox!

Energy mastery is about remaining open and continually learning and growing. Life offers never-ending learning and growth. Now that you are aligned you must continue to challenge yourself in new ways.

> *"If you're not growing, you're dying."*
>
> William S. Burroughs

Now there's nothing wrong with dying but if you are living, I invite you to notice when you learn something new and try to learn something new every single day. Neuroplasticity is a fairly recent scientific discovery that your brain is moldable and growable. I touched briefly on this book about neural pathways and how your habits live in the grooves of those pathways and how you can create new ones over time. What inroads are you making inside of your head? What are some things you would like to learn? It could be anything at all from business and marketing skills to gardening, cooking, learning to fly a plane, or surf. Anything at all! You get to choose! How incredible is that? Life is an epic adventure. Never give up.

Conclusion

Congratulations! From your foundation to embodiment and ongoing maintenance, you now have the awareness, tools, and knowledge to live a life of energy mastery! If you've made it this far in the book you are amazing and one of the few who reads a whole book. Congratulations! Have a celebratory dance party!

What I hope you've gained from reading this book is that you, your TRUE SELF, are connected to the greatest force in the universe, Divine Love. Even if you haven't felt it or exercised it in the past, you can live your life connected to this power. When you do, you experience more joy, peace, and ultimate happiness. This is energy mastery.

Regardless of what you have been through or where you are now you can free yourself from the past, be empowered in the present, and courageously create your future!

Deeply consider your intentions for your life, and as you begin declaring them watch as seeming obstacles are moved miraculously, or you find the solution to move ahead within yourself.

Drop into your heart every day and connect deeply with your true self and your vision for your life. Take actions and make choices from this place of visionary connection.

If you have read this book and are on your path, no other choice will suffice. Living out of integrity is no longer an option, and that is greatness. After you put this book down, live from a place of self-awareness and curiosity.

My friend Lindsay Umlah said it best, "Curiosity is gonna save the world!"

This journey of life isn't over yet. Each day is a fresh opportunity to love yourself and others openly and freely. Create what you came here to create and give it your all; whatever that means to you.

Remember you can choose and create happiness. Set up those triggers in your life by anchoring them in with enthusiasm. Have reminders around you in your environment, whether sticky notes on mirrors or reminders on your phone. Be gently aware of your lovely lizard brain which will try to keep you 'safe', when you are already safe. Remember, you can tell it "thank you for sharing" and choose to act anyway, one step at a time.

Remember to breathe and relax, feel into your own body on all levels; mental, emotional, physical, and spiritual. Be willing to forgive and let go, put a smile on your face, surround yourself with like-minded people, and get help when you need it. You are not meant to do this alone.

From my heart to yours, I wish you truth and kindness in the way of energy mastery.

XO
Vicki

The 10 Commandments of Energy Mastery

1. Cultivate Gentle Awareness

2. Nourish Thyself

3. Love Thyself

4. Follow Thy Heart

5. Own our Boundaries

6. Love Your Body

7. Breathe and Meditate

8. Forgive and Let Go

9. Take Action

10. Never Give Up

About the Author

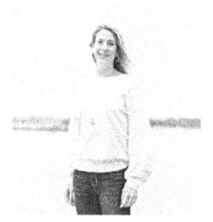

Vicki Adrianne is a powerhouse spiritual healer and coach. Vicki Knows that whatever you have been through, you can heal and learn the lessons of your past and she hopes this book gives you courage and skills to rise.

Vicki serves those who have had their spiritual awakening through one-on-one and small group programs to help them let go of what keeps them stuck and distrusting so they can access true inner freedom and authentic personal power. She is the creator of the courses "Let Go and Live On!" and "Clear Confidence Energy Mastery". Her other books include "Connect, Strengthen, Surrender", and "Woman Rise".

Learn more at www.VickiAdrianne.com

www.ingramcontent.com/pod-product-compliance
Lightning Source LLC
Chambersburg PA
CBHW071810080526
44589CB00012B/746